Mayo Clinic Guide

DATE DUE

DEC 1 4 2009			
DEC 0 4 2017			

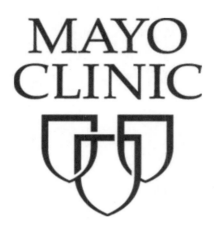

Mayo Clinic Guide
to Living with
a Spinal Cord Injury

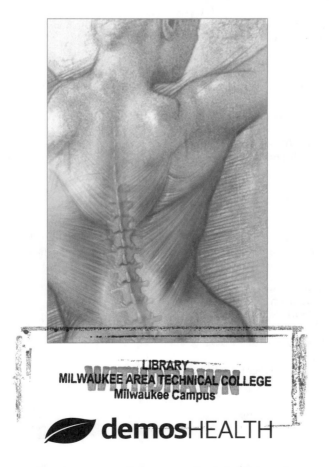

demosHEALTH

Visit our web site at www.demosmedpub.com

Medical information provided by Demos Health, in the absence of a visit with a health-care professional, must be considered as an educational service only. This book is not designed to replace a physician's independent judgment about the appropriateness or risks of a procedure or therapy for a given patient. Our purpose is to provide you with information that will help you make your own health-care decisions.

The information and opinions provided here are believed to be accurate and sound, based on the best judgment available to the authors, editors, and publisher, but readers who fail to consult appropriate health authorities assume the risk of any injuries. The authors, editors, and publisher are not responsible for errors or omissions. The editors and publisher welcome any reader to report to the publisher any discrepancies or inaccuracies noticed.

Library of Congress Cataloging-in-Publication Data
Mayo clinic guide to living with a spinal cord injury.
     p. cm.
  Includes index.
  ISBN-13: 978-1-932603-77-4 (pbk. : alk. paper)
  ISBN-10: 1-932603-77-8 (pbk. : alk. paper)
  1. Spinal cord—Wounds and injuries.
  RD594.3.M39 2009
  617.4'82044—dc22

                    2009005186

Special discounts on bulk quantities of Demos Medical Publishing books are available to corporations, professional associations, pharmaceutical companies, health care organizations, and other qualifying groups. For details, please contact:

Special Sales Department
Demos Medical Publishing
386 Park Avenue South, Suite 301
New York, NY 10016
Phone: 800–532–8663 or 212–683–0072
Fax: 212–683–0118
E-mail: orderdept@demosmedpub.com

Made in the United States of America

09 10 11 12   5 4 3 2 1

Contents

Foreword

If you are reading this book, more than likely your life has been in some way affected by spinal cord injury (SCI). Perhaps you have sustained such an injury, or possibly someone close to you. Regardless, becoming knowledgeable about managing the consequences of the injury is essential. The knowledge imparted in this book will help restore your hope for the future.

No doubt, life is changed when one sustains a spinal cord injury. The injury will likely place tremendous strains upon one's physical health, emotional health, relationships, career, finances, and a host of other life domains. People with spinal cord injuries and their families often become so overwhelmed that the best they can hope for is survival.

This book is not about merely surviving a spinal cord injury—it provides fundamental information necessary to thrive following an injury.

In the 15 years since I sustained my spinal cord injury, I have never been more positive that the future holds hope for people with spinal cord injuries. No society has ever been more accommodating to life with SCI. Medical advances and rehabilitation techniques have never been able to restore greater levels of independence to people with spinal cord injury. Research has never been closer to a cure for SCI.

This book will assist you to maximize your independence and quality of life following SCI—use it wisely and never lose hope in your future.

Paul J. Tobin
President
United Spinal Association

Preface

A spinal cord injury or disease can have dramatic effects on the person affected and his or her family. However, coordinated teamwork by nurses, therapists, technicians, psychologists, physicians and surgeons can help a person with a spinal cord injury return to the highest level of activity possible. Ongoing research continues to reveal new interventions and treatments, and today people with spinal cord injury recover more completely than any time in history. However, changes in the U.S. health care system have made it more challenging to provide all the information needed. Because hospital stays are now quite compressed in comparison to the past, time spent in the hospital is short, hectic and exhausting. For dozens of years, the material presented in this book has been the foundation of our educational program for patients. In recent years we've found that it's much more difficult for us to deliver and for patients to embrace the educational material due to short hospital stays. This change was necessary, but it places the educational needs of patients and their families in jeopardy. Therefore, we hope the publication of the educational material in this book will help people with spinal cord injury advocate for their needs, proactively manage their health and partner with health care providers to enhance and maintain their wellness.

Mayo Clinic is a large multi-specialty healthcare delivery system that is built upon an integrated model of care, teamwork, research and education. Mayo Clinic's primary value is "The needs of the patient come first." Over the last 40 years Mayo Clinic has served individuals with spinal cord disorders through its coordinated spinal cord injury program. Throughout the history of the program patient education has been of paramount importance. The material presented in this book represents the collective work of the therapists, nurses, psychologists, physicians and educators who wrote and revised it for the benefit of the patients they served. Because hundreds of Mayo Clinic staff members have contributed to this book, individual authors are not listed. This book is the product of interdisciplinary teamwork, one of the hallmarks of Mayo Clinic care. Additionally, feedback from our patients and their evolving needs over time have shaped the content and guided countless revisions of the material presented in this book. We owe thanks to all the patients who have provided feedback over the years.

The topics presented in this book may raise additional questions. The final section of the book contains resources that may be helpful in answering those questions. Clinicians specializing in spinal cord injury are also an important source of information, especially because new information is continually available. These clinicians can be found in specialized spinal cord injury centers around the world. State, national and international organizations focused on spinal cord care are also an important source for new information. The content of this book is the basic material many people with a spinal cord injury or disease need to know. The utility of the information we present in this book has been tested and used for years and our patients have told us it is helpful. We hope you will find it useful as well. New innovations in care are constantly being developed and many of the web sites listed at the end of the book are excellent resources for "cutting edge" information.

This preface would be incomplete without highlighting Dr. Joachim Optiz for his pioneering leadership of the Mayo Clinic Spinal Cord Injury Program in its formative years. He led the initial efforts to write and systematically update early versions of this book. His attention to detail, inquisitive spirit and dedication to patient care built the foundation of our program and we are the beneficiaries of his creative vision.

Ronald K. Reeves, MD
Medical Director, Spinal Cord Injury Program
Vice Chair, Department of Physical Medicine and Rehabilitation
Mayo Clinic
Rochester, Minnesota, USA

Mayo Clinic Guide to Living with a Spinal Cord Injury

I

Living with Spinal Cord Injury

1 Introduction to Spinal Cord Injury

An injury or disease affecting the spinal cord causes a major life change. Such an injury or disease raises many questions, concerns and fears about the present and the future. In dealing with these concerns, you will need advice and information. Talking and listening to caregivers can help. Your efforts to learn about your condition and the challenges you will face are especially important.

This chapter will explain:
- What spinal cord injury (SCI)/dysfunction is
- Effects of SCI on body function
- Changes in body function and how to adapt and manage
- Some changes you may face and how to cope with them

You and your family's active involvement in learning about all aspects of SCI is the key to a successful rehabilitation program. Definitions of terms you may not be familar with are provided in the glossary.

THE REHABILITATION HEALTH CARE TEAM

During your rehabilitation, a team of many health professionals will be involved in your care. The team may meet regularly with you and your family to set rehabilitation goals, review your progress, update your program, and plan for your return to the community.

Members of this team include:

You and Your Family Members

You, the patient, and your family are the most important members of the rehabilitation team. Active participation by you and your family in planning goals and therapy is key to effective rehabilitation. With your permission, the rehabilitation team shares progress assessments with family members involved in your care so that they understand overall progress, expectations for further rehabilitation and discharge goals.

Physiatrists

Physiatrists are physicians who specialize in physical medicine and rehabilitation, and are responsible for your overall medical care. They coordinate rehabilitation therapies, services, and the care you require from other physicians.

Psychologists

Rehabilitation psychologists are trained in the psychology of adjustment to disability. They have a Ph.D. and are credentialed by the American Board of Rehabilitation Psychology. Rehabilitation psychologists assess how you are coping. They work with you and your family, and other members of the rehabilitation team to help you adjust to your disability and plan for the future. Frequent areas of intervention include stress management, coping with loss, sexuality, and vocational planning.

Rehabilitation Nurses

The nursing staff includes registered nurses (RNs) who have specialized education in spinal cord rehabilitation, licensed practical nurses and patient care assistants. Rehabilitation RNs assess your ongoing psychosocial status, physical adjustment and progress with functional rehabilitation. Nursing staff assist with all aspects of your care, including preventive respiratory care, bowel and bladder management, and both therapeutic and preventive skin care. The RN's primary goal is teaching you about spinal cord injury, how to direct others in your care and how to be as independent as possible. The RN works with other members of your health care team in discharge planning and coordinating your transition to the next level of care.

Physical Therapists

SCI causes weakness, incoordination, and fatigue. A physical therapist helps you regain muscle function, increase mobility and learn how to use the appropriate adaptive equipment. Physical therapists have specialized expertise in wheelchairs and functional electrical stimulation.

Occupational Therapists

Occupational therapists help you develop the functional abilities needed in daily life, such as self-care and home management. Occupational therapists also address swallowing, upper extremity functioning, cognition and safety, and visual perception. Occupational therapists have special expertise in wheelchairs, rehabilitation after upper extremity functional restoration surgery, and driving after SCI.

Respiratory Therapists and Respiratory Therapy Technicians

If your spinal cord injury involves the neck or upper back, you may have difficulty coughing effectively. If you have cervical injuries affecting C1–C4 vertebrae, you may also have difficulty breathing. Respiratory therapists evaluate, treat and care for patients with breathing disorders, and are responsible for respiratory care treatments. If you require a ventilator to breathe after SCI, respiratory therapists help ensure that you, as well as your family, friends or support system, know how to use the ventilator.

Recreational Therapists

A critical part of recovery after SCI is the ability to return to social, family and recreational activities. In many instances, SCI changes how someone can participate in hobbies and family activities. A recreational therapist will help you adjust to the hobbies and activities you participated in before your injury, to develop new skills and interests, and get involved in the community through re-integration trips. Recreational therapists provide opportunities to apply learned skills from other therapies to leisure activities.

Speech-Language Pathologists

Some spinal cord injuries can affect speech, or may occur with a brain injury. In these situations speech-language pathologists will evaluate speech and language abilities. The speech pathologist assists with the skills necessary for communication, or possibly develops alternative methods of communication. Speech therapists are also trained in day-to-day interventions and training to improve communication.

Social Workers

Medical social workers can assist you and your family in various ways, by counseling you and your loved ones, providing emotional support, and offering information about financial resources and community agencies.

Chaplains

Caring for your spiritual needs is very important. Chaplains provide spiritual or religious support for you and your family throughout the recovery process.

Dietitians

Adequate nutrition is critical to recovery after SCI. A registered dietitian can help you make healthy food choices and to manage any special dietary needs you may have.

EFFECTS OF SPINAL CORD INJURY

Your spinal cord may be damaged by injury (motor vehicle crash, fall, sporting accident), or disease (infection, tumors, blood clots). When your spinal cord is damaged, your body may not function as it did. Messages to and from the brain may not be able to pass through the damaged area of your spinal cord.

Normal Anatomy and Function of the Spinal Cord

The central nervous system consists of the brain and spinal cord. The spinal cord extends downward from the base of your brain and is made up of nerve cells and groups of nerves called tracts, which go to different parts of your body. The lower end of your spinal cord stops a little above your waist in a region called the conus medullaris. Below this region is a group of nerve roots called the cauda equina. (Figure 1).

Your spinal cord is enclosed in a fluid-filled sac called the thecal sac. The fluid inside this sac is spinal fluid. The thecal sac and spinal cord are protected by the bones (vertebrae) of the spinal column (Figure 2).

Tracts in your spinal cord carry messages between the brain and the rest of the body. Motor tracts carry signals from the brain to control

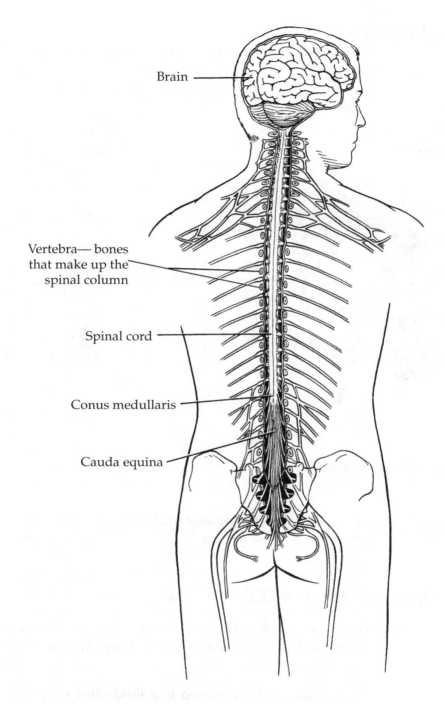

Figure 1. Central nervous system.

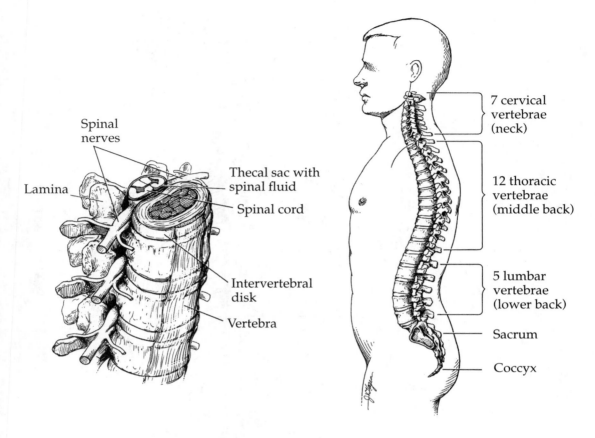

Figure 2. Spinal column.

muscle movement. Sensory tracts carry signals from body parts to the brain relating to heat, cold, pressure, pain and the position of your limbs.

Bodily Function Effects of SCI

The lowest normally functioning segment of your spinal cord is referred to as the neurologic level of your injury. If all sensory (feeling) and motor function (ability to control movement) are lost below this neurologic level, your injury is called complete. If you have some motor or sensory function below the affected area, your injury may be called incomplete. Your ability to control your limbs is determined by the level at which your spinal cord injury occurred and the degree of completeness (Figure 3). Your rehabilitation health care provider (physiatrist) will perform a series of tests to determine the level and completeness of your injury.

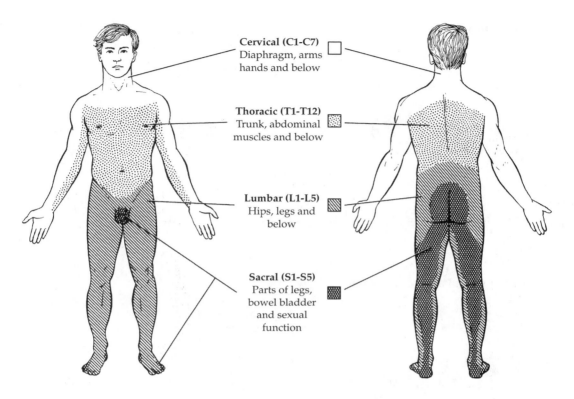

Figure 3. Neurologic level and potentially affected body parts.

Some incomplete spinal cord injuries may result in syndromes that affect sensory and/or motor function. The following are common incomplete syndromes:

- *Central cord syndrome:* Caused by damage to the central part of the spinal cord and usually involves the cervical region. It causes greater loss of function and sensation in the upper limbs than the lower limbs (Figure 4a).
- *Anterior cord syndrome:* Caused by damage to the anterior spinal artery, which supplies blood to the front of the spinal cord. The result is loss of function, pain and temperature sensation below the level of injury. However, persons with this syndrome may be able to sense the position, vibration and touch of the para- lyzed limbs (Figure 4b).
- *Brown-Séquard syndrome:* Caused by damage to one side of the spinal cord. It produces loss of function and position sense on one side of the body and a loss of pain and temperature on the opposite side of the body (Figure 4c).
- *Conus medullaris syndrome:* Caused by damage to the conus and lumbar nerve roots. It may produce flaccid bladder and

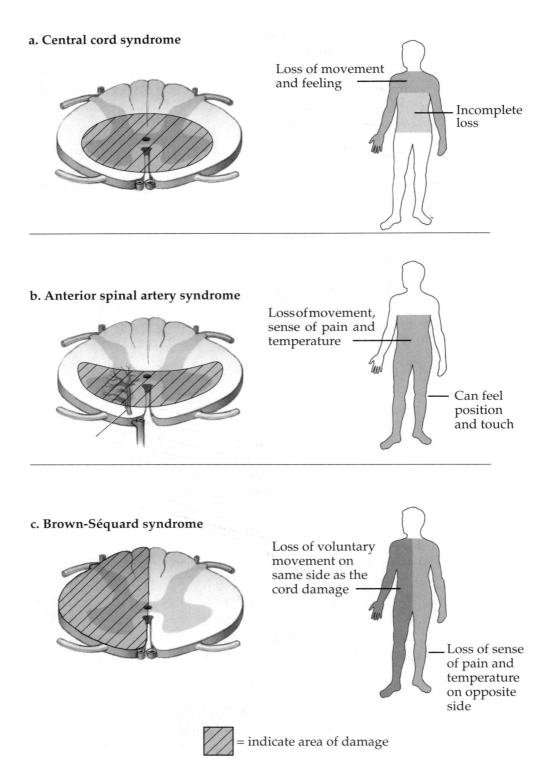

a. Central cord syndrome

Loss of movement and feeling

Incomplete loss

b. Anterior spinal artery syndrome

Loss of movement, sense of pain and temperature

Can feel position and touch

c. Brown-Séquard syndrome

Loss of voluntary movement on same side as the cord damage

Loss of sense of pain and temperature on opposite side

= indicate area of damage

Figure 4. Types of incomplete spinal cord injury syndromes.

bowel, change in sexual function, and loss of function of the lower limbs (Figure 5).

- *Cauda equina syndrome:* Caused by damage below the conus to the lumbosacral nerve roots. It may also produce flaccid bladder and bowel, change in sexual function, and loss of function of the lower limbs (Figure 5).

Physical effects of SCI

At first, changes in the way your body functions may be overwhelming. However, you can learn new skills and how to adapt old skills to deal with the physical effects of SCI.

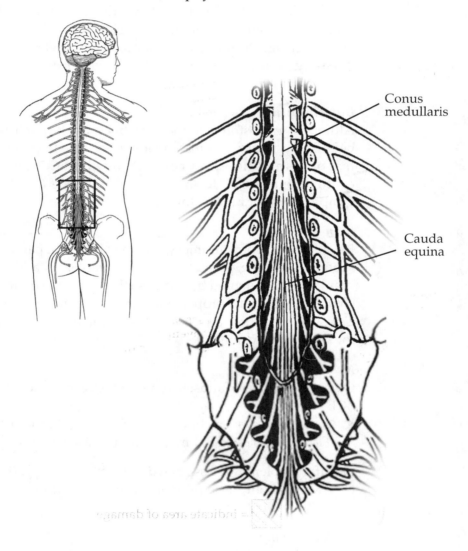

Figure 5. Conus medullaris and cauda equina of spinal cord.

Paralysis from spinal cord injury that affects your arms, trunk and legs is called **tetraplegia (quadriplegia).** Paralysis that affects all or part of the legs and all or part of your trunk is called **paraplegia**.

Respiratory system

Your injury may also affect the major muscles that help you breathe. These include the diaphragm and the muscles in your chest wall and abdomen. Your level of injury will determine if and what kind of breathing problems you may have. See *Respiratory Care*, Chapter Two for additional information.

Bladder control

Your bladder will continue to store urine from your kidneys. However, due to your SCI, you may have lost the ability to control bladder emptying. During rehabilitation, you will learn new techniques to empty your bladder. See *Bladder Management*, Chapter Two for more information.

Bowel control

Although your stomach and intestines work much like they did before your injury, you may no longer be able to control the muscle that opens and closes your anus. You will learn new techniques to control your bowel during rehabilitation. See *Bowel Management*, Chapter Two for more information.

Skin

Below the level of your injury, you may have lost part or all skin sensations. Therefore, your skin nerves cannot send a message to your brain when it is injured by things such as prolonged pressure, heat or cold. You will learn proper skin care during rehabilitation. See *Skin Care*, Chapter Three and *Body Temperature Control*, in Chapter Four, for more information.

Muscle tone

One of two types of muscle tone problems may develop following SCI:
- *Spastic muscles:* Uncontrolled tightening or motion of muscles.
- *Flaccid muscles:* Soft, limp, without muscle tone.

Specific problems are associated with both spastic and flaccid muscles. More about these problems can be found in *Muscle, Joint and Bone Changes* in Chapter Three.

Skeletal changes

Immobility (inability to move) can cause your bones to lose calcium. Loss of calcium from your bones can cause osteoporosis. This condition can weaken your bones, and they may break more easily from minor stress or injury.

If your joints are not regularly moved through their full range of motion, you may lose joint flexibility. This loss of movement can result in a contracture ("frozen" joint). Joint contractures can affect your posture while lying, sitting or standing. Therapy may help prevent joint contractures. See *Muscle, Joint and Bone Changes*, Chapter Three for more information.

Circulatory control

After spinal cord injury, there may be circulatory problems ranging from spinal shock immediately following your SCI, to orthostatic hypotension and swelling of your extremities throughout your lifetime. Changes in your circulation may place you at risk for developing deep venous thrombosis and pulmonary embolus. See *Circulatory Changes*, Chapter Four, for more information.

Another problem with circulatory control is autonomic hyperreflexia (dysreflexia), which is a potentially life-threatening rise in blood pressure and is described more in *Autonomic Hyperreflexia*, Chapter Four.

Sexual function, fertility and sexuality

Sexual function, fertility and sexuality are three distinct topics and each may be affected by your injury. These topics are addressed in *Sexual Health*, Chapter Five.

Organs not affected by SCI

The following organs are typically not affected by spinal cord injury:

Heart

Your heart continues beating to supply your body's need for blood. The heart has its own internal nerve supply. However, SCI may affect the rate of your heartbeat.

Internal organs and glands

Your liver, spleen, kidneys and major glands, such as your thyroid, pancreas and adrenal glands, should continue to function normally. These organs and glands are not controlled through the spinal cord.

Coping with spinal cord injury

SCI may be devastating and may be emotionally upsetting for you, your family and friends. Everyone will have questions. You may ask some and be afraid to ask others for fear of what the answers may be. Nevertheless, asking the tough questions helps you prepare and adjust to life with SCI.

Initially, the physical and psychological changes caused by the injury may seem overwhelming. You can learn to cope with your situation with the help of a specialized rehabilitation team. This team includes physicians, nurses, social workers, psychologists, and physical, occupational and recreational therapists. Others, such as those who have experienced SCI, are also often open to listening, empathizing, and responding to your questions knowledgeably. See *Relationships with Families and Loved Ones* and *Stress and Coping Skills*, in Chapter Seven for more information.

Managing Changes to Your Body

2 Dealing with Internal Organ Functions

RESPIRATORY CARE

You may experience changes to your respiratory system following spinal cord injury. This section will help you understand how SCI may affect your respiratory system, including ways to prevent problems, deep breathing and coughing techniques, and information about infections.

The respiratory system includes your nose, mouth, windpipe (trachea) and lungs. When you breathe, air that contains oxygen passes into your lungs, where it enters your blood, and waste products, including carbon dioxide, are removed. The major respiratory muscle used for breathing is the diaphragm (Figure 1).

The diaphragm separates the chest cavity from the abdominal cavity. As you breathe in, the diaphragm moves downward, allowing the lungs to expand. Other muscle groups such as the intercostals (between the ribs) and neck muscles also help you breathe, pulling the ribs up and out.

Membranes that line your airways moisten the air you breathe. The glands in these membranes constantly produce secretions that must be removed from time to time to prevent buildup. Coughing is an important method to remove secretions.

How SCI Affects Your Respiratory System

Following SCI, the muscles that help you to breathe and remove secretions may not function normally. The level of your SCI deter-

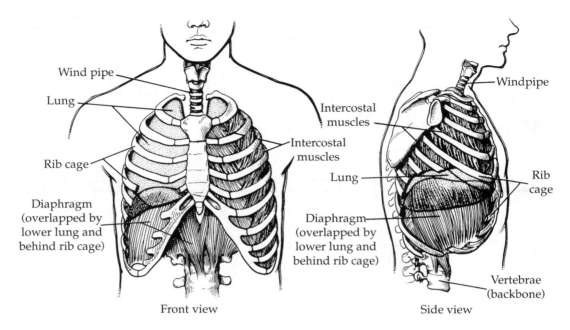

Wind pipe

Lung

Rib cage

Diaphragm
(overlapped by
lower lung and
behind rib cage)

Intercostal
muscles

Intercostal
muscles

Lung

Diaphragm
(overlapped by
lower lung and
behind rib cage)

Front view

Windpipe

Rib
cage

Vertebrae
(backbone)

Side view

Figure 1. Diaphragm.

mines which muscles are affected. Nerves at the C3 through C5 (cervical) level control your diaphragm.

Those with SCI at and above the C3 level may need a machine (such as a ventilator or breathing stimulator) to help them breathe. People with SCI at the C3 through C7 level also may require a ventilator either temporarily or permanently, since the muscles may be too weak for efficient breathing.

Respiratory muscle weakness also may be present when your injury is between the T1 through T12 (thoracic) level. Respiratory function is usually less affected with a lower level of injury. You can have normal respiratory muscle function if your injury occurred at or below the T12 level.

Depending on the level of your injury, following SCI, you may experience one or more of the following respiratory symptoms:

Muscle weakness

Persons with tetraplegia or with high-level paraplegia may note changes in breathing with different body positions. This is due to weak respiratory muscles. When lying down, the pressure of the abdominal contents on the diaphragm assists with breathing. When sitting up, an abdominal binder (corset) may help support the abdominal wall and contents by applying pressure on the diaphragm. Muscle weakness can also reduce the effectiveness of a cough's ability to move secretions and clear your lungs.

Excess secretions

Occasionally your lungs may have more secretions than usual even with regular coughing and deep breathing. These secretions, if not removed, could lead to lung infection. The most common signs of increased secretions include:
- Congestion in your chest
- Spontaneous coughing or increased need to cough
- Tickle in your throat

Hypoxia (not enough oxygen in the blood)

Hypoxia is a lack of oxygen to the body's cells. It can occur from either an inability to inhale enough oxygen, difficulty breathing, or inadequate circulation of oxygen in your bloodstream, which can occur with significant blood loss or very low hemoglobin levels.

Symptoms of hypoxia include:
- Increased rapid, shallow breathing
- Pale color
- Shortness of breath
- Increased heart rate

The treatment is oxygen provided either via nasal canula mask, tracheostomy or ventilator.

Infection

Signs of infection include:
- A change in the color of secretions
- Unusual taste of secretions
- Fever
- Shortness of breath
- Chest pain
- Cough

Without treatment, a respiratory infection can lead to pneumonia. If any of these symptoms occur, immediately contact a health care professional. Most respiratory infections can be treated with antibiotics.

Treatment and Prevention of Respiratory Problems

The highest risk of developing symptoms of a respiratory problem, such as those listed above, occurs immediately following SCI. Aggressive respiratory care is performed by nurses and respiratory therapists to prevent and treat these symptoms. As you become more active, the need for respiratory care will decrease. However, attempts to prevent respiratory problems will continue throughout your life.

Your respiratory care may include:

Tracheostomy

Some individuals require a tracheostomy in the intensive care unit to help manage secretions. A tracheostomy is a surgically created passageway between the skin of your windpipe (trachea) and neck (Figure 2). This passageway allows you to breathe more easily. The external opening in the skin is called a stoma.

Secretions may be suctioned from your tracheostomy to assist you in maintaining a clear airway. The assisted-cough technique de-

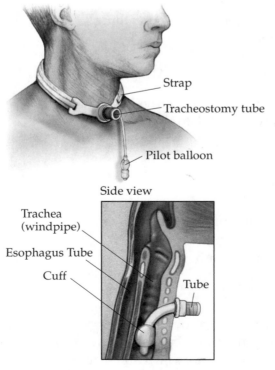

Figure 2. Tracheostomy.

scribed later in this information, may help you bring up the secretions so that they are easily suctioned.

Depending on the level of your SCI, your tracheostomy may be temporary and allowed to close when your respiratory muscles become stronger. To breathe, individuals with a SCI above C3 may require a permanent tracheostomy and a ventilator or breathing stimulator.

Deep breathing exercises

Deep breathing is important. It expands areas of the lungs that are not expanded during normal breathing. Deep breathing also causes you to cough more productively and clear secretions from your airway. Deep breathing exercises are best done lying on your back (Figures 3 and 4). They can also be done while sitting. Begin by breathing in (inhaling) as deeply as possible, pushing your abdomen outward as you breathe in. This will pull your diaphragm down. Hold your breath for 1 to 2 seconds. Then slowly let your breath out (exhale). Repeat this exercise 6 to 10 times using relaxed breathing between each exercise.

Postural drainage (bronchial drainage)

Postural drainage, also called bronchial drainage, uses gravity to help drain secretions from your lungs. Before beginning this technique, loosen any tight or restrictive clothing. Inhaler medications may be prescribed for use prior to the treatment. The medication can help to relax and open the airways in your lungs. If you can, be

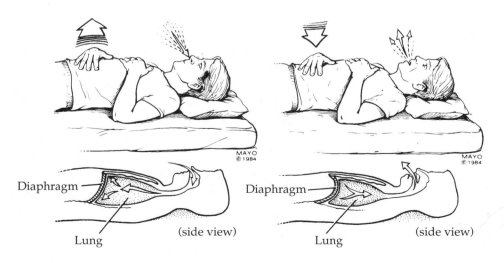

Figure 3. Breathing in.   **Figure 4.** Breathing out.

positioned so that your head is lower than your hips. Stay in one position for at least 15 minutes and then move to another position. For example, lie on your right side for 15 minutes, then on your left side for 15 minutes, or on your stomach for 15 minutes, and then on your left side for 15 minutes, etc. Use deep breathing techniques before and during bronchial drainage.

Percussion (chest clapping)

Percussion is a rapid alternating clapping of the chest wall (over the ribs) with cupped hands. It helps loosen secretions through vibration while you are in the bronchial drainage position. Someone else will have to do the chest clapping for you. A folded bath towel can be placed over the area being clapped to prevent skin irritation. You should be positioned on each side for 5 to 10 minutes during the procedure. Breathe deeply and cough during the drainage and chest clapping on each side.

Coughing exercises

Coughing helps prevent secretion buildup in your lungs. Coughing exercises are done with deep breathing exercises while lying on your back. In that position, you can cough stronger and breathe deeper. Take a deep breath, hold it for 1 to 2 seconds, and then cough. The force of a cough is normally produced by contraction of the abdominal muscles. If your abdominal muscles are paralyzed or weak, you may need assistance coughing.

Assisted-cough technique

To perform the assisted-cough technique, lie with a firm surface behind the trunk of your body and make sure your head is supported. Elevate your head if possible. Ask your caregiver to place the heel of his or her hand midway between your umbilicus (belly button) and xiphoid process (bottom of your breastbone). Breathe deeply and then exhale. As you exhale, the caregiver should give a rapid and forceful inward and slightly upward thrust toward the chest with the heel of his or her hand. This may need to be repeated several times.

Nebulized bronchodilating medications

Nebulized bronchodilating medications may be prescribed to expand your airways and assist with breathing. It helps to use this medication prior to the treatments mentioned above. Talk to your health care provider to determine if nebulized bronchodilating medications are appropriate for you.

Respiratory devices

Respiratory devices can also be used to help with deep breathing exercises. One device is the incentive spirometer, which encourages deep breathing and has a mouthpiece through which you inhale (Figure 5). In addition, other respiratory devices may be recommended to assist with lung expansion and to help loosen secretions.

Sleep apnea

Sleep apnea is a disorder characterized by frequent, brief pauses in breathing during sleep, resulting in reduced oxygen flow to the

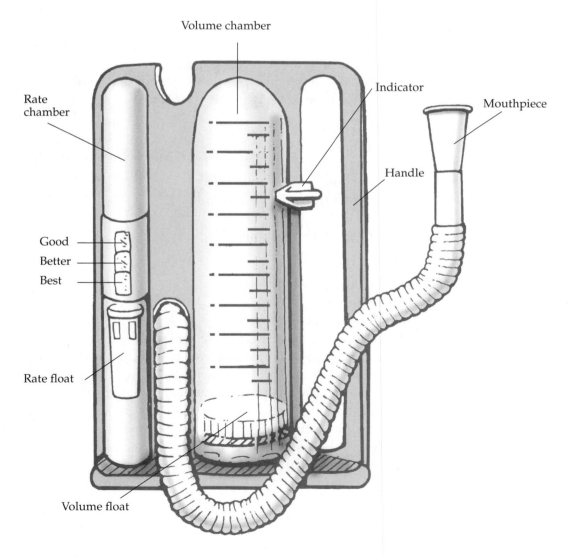

Figure 5. The incentive spirometer.

brain. While the disorder occurs in 4 percent of the general population, sleep apnea is significantly more common in persons with SCI, especially those with tetraplegia. Several factors may contribute to this higher prevalence. Obesity is relatively common in the SCI population, and individuals with SCI are predominantly males. Both are known risk factors for sleep apnea in the general population.

Weakness of respiratory muscles may contribute to sleep apnea. If you have tetraplegia, the muscles cannot easily interrupt episodes of apnea. Persons with tetraplegia often rely on neck and upper chest muscles to help with breathing because the diaphragm muscle may not have normal strength. Medications that may cause sedation are also considered potential risk factors because these drugs can slow breathing.

Additionally, lying on your back while sleeping can increase episodes of sleep apnea in the non-SCI population. Many individuals with SCI are unable to change position while in bed, which may result in increased time spent lying on your back.

Symptoms of sleep apnea include:
- Loud snoring
- Pauses in breathing during sleep
- Shortness of breath upon awakening
- Dry mouth and throat in the morning
- Morning headache
- Daytime fatigue and sleepiness
- Difficulty concentrating

Treatment for sleep apnea includes:
- Weight reduction
- Sleeping on your side
- CPAP (continuous positive airway pressure) device—During sleep, a face or nasal mask is connected to a pump that forces air into the nasal passages at pressures high enough to overcome obstructions in the airway and stimulate normal breathing. The airway pressure delivered into the upper airway is continuous during inhaling and exhaling. CPAP is safe and effective, even for children. Daytime sleepiness, heart function and hypertension may improve with CPAP use. Most importantly, quality of life may also improve.
- BiPAP (Biphasic positive airway pressure)—Pressure-controlled ventilation allows unrestricted spontaneous breathing during the entire respiratory cycle. In BiPAP, high and low airway pressures are adjusted to optimize inhalation and exhalation.

Obstructed Airway

If you have swallowing difficulties, your caregiver must know what to do for an obstructed airway. He or she should know how to perform the assisted-cough technique, the Heimlich maneuver and cardiopulmonary resuscitation (CPR).

If you are choking and no one is around, you may be able to clear your airway by doing abdominal thrusts on yourself. To do abdominal thrusts, place your fists on the soft area between your belly button and breastbone and push up forcefully. If this does not work, quickly lean forward throwing yourself onto your thighs. If this does not clear your airway, immediately get assistance.

Life Long Respiratory Health

Keeping your lungs healthy requires life-long prevention of respiratory problems and infections.
- Practice deep breathing and coughing exercises twice daily.
- Do not smoke.
- Do not expose yourself to secondhand smoke.
- Avoid large crowds during the flu season.
- Avoid people with colds.
- Keep your immunizations current.
- Practice good hand washing.
- Stay well hydrated.

Smoking reduces the efficiency of the respiratory system. It increases production of secretions in your lungs. It also damages airway linings, decreasing your ability to clear secretions from your lungs.

Keep current with immunizations for respiratory infections. These include the vaccine for pneumonia, which you should get every five years, and the flu vaccine, which is available every year.

BLADDER MANAGEMENT

Spinal cord injury can affect the function of the urinary system and may result in loss of bladder control and urinary tract complications. These conditions may be temporary or permanent and can also occur over time. This section discusses some changes in urinary function that may follow SCI and how to manage these changes.

Function of Your Urinary System

How the urinary system normally works

The urinary system includes the kidneys, ureters, bladder and urethra. Urine is produced by your kidneys and consists of water and waste products that the kidneys removed from your blood. From the kidneys, urine travels down two long muscular tubes called ureters to the bladder (Figure 6).

Your bladder is a hollow muscular organ that stores urine. The pelvic floor muscles help to hold urine in the bladder. They surround the urethra, rectum and vagina (in women). The urethra is a tube leading from your bladder to the outside of your body. Urine passes through the ureters, then the bladder and exits the body through the urethra. The muscle that surrounds the urethra is called the external urethral sphincter. This muscle and the base of the bladder (bladder neck) form the urinary outlet (Figures 7 and 8).

Normally, bladder function is controlled by voiding centers in the brain and the spinal cord. While the bladder is filling with urine,

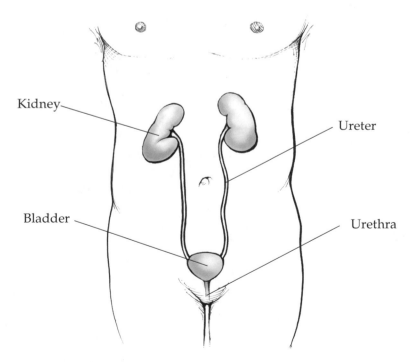

Figure 6. The urinary system.

the voiding centers keep the bladder muscle (detrusor muscle) relaxed and the pelvic floor muscles, including the urethral sphincter muscle, tense. This holds urine in the bladder. When the bladder is full and you decide to urinate (void), the voiding centers signal the bladder muscle to contract, causing the bladder neck to open and form a funnel (Figure 9). The pelvic floor muscles, including the urethral sphincter, relax and urine flows out of the urethra.

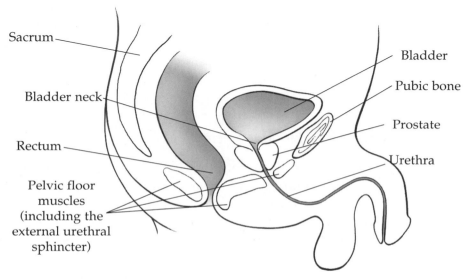

Figure 7. Male lower urinary system.

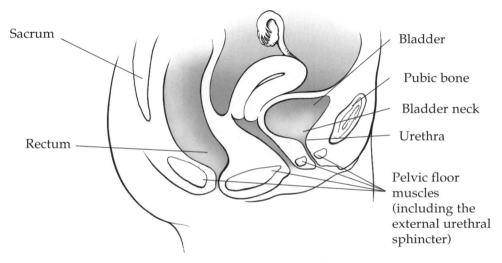

Figure 8. Female lower urinary system.

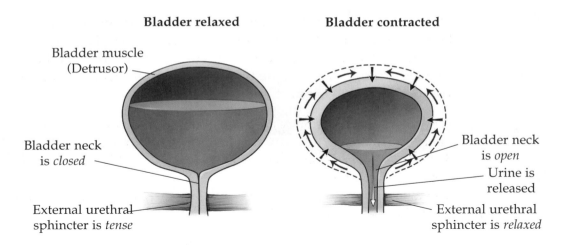

Figure 9. Bladder function.

Changes in bladder function

Nerve centers in the brain and the spinal cord are important to urination (voiding). Communication between these nerve centers occurs through long nerve fibers that run the length of the spinal cord. SCI can affect this communication and therefore, problems with urine storage and bladder emptying may result. Injury to the spinal cord can result in changes in:

- The ability to sense when your bladder is full.
- Your ability to empty your bladder on your own.
- The tone (muscle tension and responsiveness) and your control of the pelvic floor (outlet) muscles.
- The tone of the bladder muscle.

Pre-existing conditions such as an overstretched bladder, enlarged prostate (in men), weak pelvic floor muscles, or previous bladder or urinary outlet surgery, can also affect bladder function.

Common bladder disorders

The location and extent of injury to your spinal cord influence changes in your bladder function. When the upper portions of the spinal cord (cervical and thoracic regions) are affected, you may develop an upper motor neuron bladder (often called a reflex or spastic bladder). Typically, the bladder tone is increased, which results in less storage capacity, an urge to urinate more often, and a sudden urge to urinate. Loss of bladder control (incontinence) can result. Since the outlet (sphincter) muscles may be spastic, incomplete bladder emptying or an interrupted urine stream may occur. Detrusor-sphincter dyssynergia occurs when the bladder muscle contracts at the same time as the outlet muscles, resulting in ineffective emptying and increased bladder pressures that can damage your kidneys.

When the lower portions of the spinal cord (lumbar and sacral regions) are affected, you may develop a lower motor neuron bladder (often called an areflexic or flaccid bladder). Bladder tone is decreased, which can cause increased storage capacity, inability to urinate, or incomplete bladder emptying. Incontinence can occur when the outlet muscles lack tone.

The region affected by your SCI cannot predict your bladder disorder with 100 percent accuracy. Several tests can help to clarify your specific bladder dysfunction and guide your bladder management options.

Measuring Your Urinary System Function

The following tests are most commonly done to find out how well your urinary system is functioning and to plan an effective bladder management program. Some tests may be done within the first year of injury. They may be repeated periodically to monitor changes in bladder function and to confirm that your bladder management program is optimal.

Urinalysis

A sample of your urine is tested to see if you have a bladder or kidney infection or other conditions.

Urine culture and bacterial sensitivity test

A urine culture shows whether your bladder or kidneys contain harmful bacteria. If you have an infection, a bacterial sensitivity test is done to determine the effectiveness of various antibiotics in destroying the bacteria and which antibiotic works best.

Renal (kidney) clearance tests

A renal clearance test shows how well your kidneys clean wastes from your blood. A substance (iothalamate or inulin) is injected into your bloodstream. After set amounts of time, small amounts of urine and blood are collected to measure how much of the substance your kidneys have filtered.

Creatinine clearance test

The creatinine clearance test is similar to the renal clearance test. However, nothing is injected into your bloodstream. Creatinine is a protein made by your muscles and filtered by your kidneys. It can help assess renal function. The test requires that you collect all of your urine for 24 hours. This test is not as accurate as the renal clearance test.

Urodynamic study (UDS)

The UDS test identifies the relationship between the bladder and the outlet. During the test, a thin, flexible tube (catheter) is passed into your bladder through the urethra. Sterile fluid is passed through this tube to fill your bladder, simulating normal filling of the bladder with urine. This part of the test helps determine how much urine your bladder can hold and how much pressure your bladder develops during filling, urine storage, and emptying (voiding) attempts.

External sphincter electromyogram (EMG)

This test shows how well your pelvic floor muscles work. Small sensors (tape electrodes) are placed on your skin over the pelvic floor. A recording shows when muscle contractions begin and end. It also shows how much the muscles contract and relax when the bladder fills and empties, and whether any voluntary muscle control occurs.

Video urodynamic study

During this study, (also called video-flow or video fluoroscopy), your bladder is filled via catheter with fluid that can be seen on X-rays. The activity of your bladder, bladder neck and pelvic floor, is monitored during filling and emptying of the bladder.

Precaution: Pregnant women should not have a video urodynamic study.

Cystoscopy

During a cystoscopy, a small tube (cystoscope) with a light on the end is inserted through the urethra into the bladder. A urologist can see the lining of your bladder, urethra and prostate (in men). Foreign bodies, such as bladder stones and cancerous tissue, can also be identified and sometimes removed during the test.

Renal (kidney) scans

These scans, using ultrasound, X-rays or computed tomography (CT), monitor kidney function and outline the shape of the kidneys, ureters and bladder. They may also be used to check for bladder and kidney stones.

Bladder Management Program

A bladder management program can help you control changes in bladder and urinary function. Such a program may also help you regularly and completely empty your bladder, and avoid pressure injury to your kidneys, incontinence and urinary tract complications. Your program may change over time, based on the changes in the health and function of your urinary system.

A bladder management program is important because it may:
- Preserve kidney function
- Prevent bladder and kidney infections
- Prevent bladder and kidney stones
- Prevent incontinence
- Maintain acceptable bladder volumes less than 400 to 500 cubic centimeters (cc), or less than two cups

Bladder management methods include:
- Continuous catheter drainage
- Intermittent catheterization
- Catheter-free voiding
- Bladder retraining

Your bladder management program is based on the method that suits you best. Sometimes, management methods may be combined. Factors such as travel, the availability and accessibility of bathrooms/toilets, or changes in your condition may require changes in your management program. Record keeping, medications, and medical or surgical procedures also may be included in your bladder management program.

Continuous catheter drainage

A catheter is placed and remains in your bladder to continuously drain urine. The catheter may be placed in the bladder through the urethra (indwelling urethra catheter) or through the abdominal wall (suprapubic catheter). With continuous catheter drainage, you must drink 2½ to 3 quarts (80 to 96 ounces or 10 to 12 glasses) of liquid per day. Liquids include beverages, such as water, and foods with high water content, such as Jell-O™, ice cream, soup and watermelon. The resulting high urine output will help flush bacteria and sediment out of your bladder.

Intermittent catheterization

Intermittent catheterization refers to the scheduled emptying of your bladder with a catheter. A thin tube is inserted through the urethra and into your bladder. Urine drains from the bladder through the tube. When your bladder is empty, the catheter is removed. Catheterization is done every four to six hours throughout the day.

To maintain acceptable bladder volumes, you will need to balance your fluid intake with your emptying (catheterization) schedule. If you drink a set amount of liquid on a regular schedule, your bladder should fill at regular times. To start, your recommended fluid intake schedule should be between 1,800 to 2,000 cc of fluid (about 60 ounces) in 24 hours.

The fluid amounts should be spread out as follows:

Time	Amount
8 a.m. (breakfast)	350 cc—about 1½ cups (12 ounces)
10 a.m.	250 cc—about 1 cup (8 ounces)
Noon (lunch)	350 cc—about 1½ cups (12 ounces)
2 p.m.	250 cc—about 1 cup (8 ounces)
4 p.m.	250 cc—about 1 cup (8 ounces)
6 p.m. (dinner)	350 cc—about 1½ cups (12 ounces)

Drink only at scheduled times during the day and take only sips after your evening meal. This schedule may be changed based on your urine output patterns or other needs.

Factors in your catheterization program may be individualized according to the technique you learn and your equipment used.

Catheter free voiding

Catheter free voiding refers to the scheduled emptying of your bladder using a voiding technique instead of a catheter. This method requires that you be able to consistently empty your bladder each time you void. Empty is defined as having less than 100 cc to 150 cc (ideally less than 50 cc) of urine left in your bladder after voiding.

Key times to void when using this method are:
• When you awaken

- An hour after your mealtime fluids
- Every two to three hours during the day
- Before you go to sleep

Balancing your fluid intake and voiding on a schedule will help you maintain acceptable bladder volumes and continence (ability to control bladder).

Bladder retraining

Bladder retraining involves learning one or more voiding techniques. For example, some techniques contract your bladder muscle, whereas others require that you use controlled force to push urine out of the bladder. In certain cases, you may learn to relax the pelvic floor muscles including the urethral sphincter muscle. When practicing the method best for you:
- Set aside enough time (about 10 minutes) so you do not feel hurried.
- Do not get discouraged. Being able to empty your bladder at regularly scheduled times takes practice.

Recording fluid intake and output

Measure and record your fluid intake and output on the bladder record. See Record of Bladder Retraining on page 34. Keeping this record is important.

Here is how you should fill in the columns of the bladder record:

Column 1:   Record the time of fluid intake.
Column 2:   Record the amount of fluid intake next to the time.
Column 3:   Record the amount of controlled (intentional) voiding and the time it occurred.
Column 4:   Record the amount of urine obtained using your voiding method.
Column 5:   Record the grade (see grade levels below) of urinary incontinence and the time the incontinence occurred. If you are using an external catheter, measure and record the amount of incontinence.
              Grade 1:   Underwear/pad is damp.
              Grade 2:   Underwear/pad is wet enough that you are thinking about changing it.
              Grade 3:   Underwear/pad and outer clothing are so wet that you must change all clothing.
              Grade 4:   Large amounts of urine leak through your clothing.

Column 6:   Record the amount of urine you obtain by catheterization. If you are retraining, this is the amount of urine remaining in your bladder after voiding (residual urine volume).

Record of Bladder Retraining

Date_____Name_____

Fluid intake (cc)		Fluid Output (cc)			
1) Time	2) All beverages; includes water, soups, ice cream, Jell-O™	3) Normal voiding (not triggered, strained or manually expressed)	4) Voiding that is triggered, strained or manually expressed	5) Incontinence or spontaneous voiding (grade level)	6) Amount of urine obtained by catheterization after voiding
1 a.m.					
2					
3					
4					
5					
6					
7					
8					
9					
10					
11					
12					
1 p.m.					
2					
3					
4					
5					
6					
7					
8					
9					
10					
11					
12					
Subtotal					
Total in		Total out			

Medications

Medications may increase the effectiveness of your bladder management program. Medications may be used alone or in combination with others, depending on changes in the function of your bladder and urinary outlet. Because these medications may have side effects, use them only as directed by your health care provider. Many over-the-counter and prescription medications can affect bladder function. Ask your health care provider for more information about the effect of these medications.

Table 1 lists some commonly used medications, their purposes and possible side effects.

Antibiotics may also be used to prevent urinary tract infections or to treat urinary tract infections.

Table 1 Medications

Drugs that	Reason for use	Possible side effects
Relax bladder tone Oxybutynin chloride (Ditropan™) Tolterodine tartrate (Detrol™)	Increase storage capacity Decrease bladder spasticity/ contractions Lower bladder pressures which are too high Decrease irritability of the bladder when a continuous drainage catheter is in place Decrease incontinence	Dry eyes Dry mouth Constipation
Relax outlet resistance Tamsulosin hydrochloride (Flomax™)	Improve emptying by decreasing tone in the bladder neck area	Low blood pressure Light-headedness Fatigue A change in ejaculation (men) Abdominal cramps

Common Urinary Tract Problems

Some common urinary tract problems may include:
- Urinary incontinence
- Bladder and/or kidney infection
- Bladder and/or kidney stones
- High pressure bladder

To help prevent urinary tract complications you should:
- Follow your bladder management program
- Keep anal and genital areas clean and dry
- Get prompt treatment for symptomatic bladder infections
- Report changes in your bladder function to your health care provider and obtain follow-up care as recommended
- Take prescribed medication as directed

Urinary incontinence

Urinary incontinence (inability to control urination) can result from a SCI. It may also result from a bladder infection or bladder stone(s). Incontinence increases the risk of skin irritation and potential skin breakdown. People who have urinary incontinence can keep their clothing dry by using an external collection device. Other products available include a variety of protective garments and pads. You can reduce your chance of incontinence by:
- Maintaining a regular drinking and bladder emptying schedule
- Preventing bladder and kidney infections

Bladder infection

A bladder infection occurs when bacteria enter the bladder and multiply. The most common causes of repeated infections are poor hygiene, incomplete bladder emptying, the presence of a foreign object in the bladder (for example, a bladder stone or catheter) and not completing antibiotic treatment for a previous infection.

Unless you experience symptoms such as those below, urine testing and antibiotic treatment are not recommended:
- Urine with a strong or unusual odor
- Cloudy or reddish-brown urine
- An urge to urinate more often than usual
- Sudden urge to urinate
- Lower abdominal pain or cramping (may not be evident if you have a lack of sensation)
- Burning sensation when urinating (may not be evident if you have a lack of sensation)
- Low energy, feeling tired or mildly ill
- Incontinence
- Increase in general body spasticity (increased spasms in the body)
- Fever
- Autonomic hyperreflexia

Kidney infection

A kidney infection (pyelonephritis) occurs when bacteria enter the kidneys and multiply. Most commonly, the bacteria move from the bladder back up the ureters. When you develop a kidney infection, bacteria may also enter your bloodstream and cause a severe and potentially life-threatening illness.

Symptoms of kidney infection may include:
• High fever
• Severe headache
• Onset of midback pain (may not be evident if you have a lack of sensation)
• Increased bladder spasticity
• Chills
• Sudden stomach upset or nausea
• Autonomic hyperreflexia

Bladder stone formation

A bladder stone forms when crystals attach onto small particles of tissue, bacteria or foreign objects (such as an indwelling catheter) in the bladder. People with SCI have an increased risk of forming bladder stones. The presence of a catheter, incomplete bladder emptying, repeated urinary tract infections and higher urine calcium concentrations increase this risk. Since bladder stones may produce no outward symptoms, regular follow-up is necessary.

Symptoms of bladder stone formation may include:
• Incontinence
• Increased bladder spasticity
• Repeated bladder infections
• Blood in urine
• Uncontrolled spasticity in arms or legs
• Autonomic hyperreflexia

Kidney stone formation

Stones may form in one or both kidneys for the same reasons as bladder stones. The stones may damage the kidneys.

Symptoms of kidney stone formation may include:
• Incontinence
• Increased bladder spasticity
• Repeated bladder infections
• Blood in urine

- Uncontrolled spasticity in arms or legs
- Autonomic hyperreflexia

High pressure bladder

In the condition known as high pressure bladder, sustained pressure develops in the bladder. This condition can be found in an upper motor neurogenic (spastic) bladder with an overactive or normal outlet, and occasionally when excessive force such as pushing on the abdomen is needed to empty your bladder. In an upper motor neurogenic (spastic) bladder, the repeated contraction of the bladder muscle can lead to a stronger, thicker bladder wall. This can damage the ureteral openings at the bladder wall. When pressure in the bladder increases, urine can be forced back up (reflux) to the kidneys (Figure 10). Your kidneys are very sensitive to pressure and continued reflux can eventually damage or even destroy them.

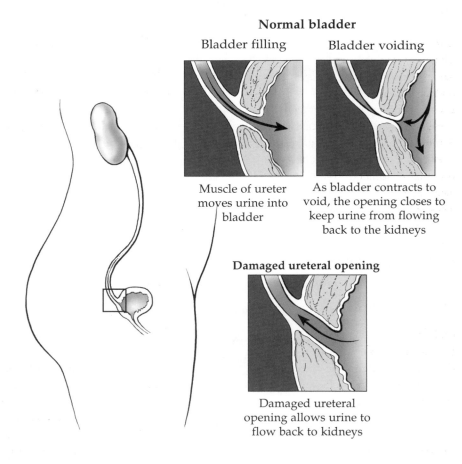

Normal bladder

Bladder filling

Bladder voiding

Muscle of ureter moves urine into bladder

As bladder contracts to void, the opening closes to keep urine from flowing back to the kidneys

Damaged ureteral opening

Damaged ureteral opening allows urine to flow back to kidneys

Figure 10. High pressure bladder.

Even if the ureteral openings are not damaged, high pressure within the bladder can impair the normal flow of urine from the kidneys. Another result might be impaired kidney function.

High bladder pressures and reflux can develop over time and occur without outward symptoms. Therefore, returning for follow-up appointments and tests is extremely important. Medications and/or procedures to decrease bladder activity, bladder pressures, or outlet resistance, may be used to preserve kidney function.

Table 2 outlines some possible urinary tract complications and how you can respond to them. Your awareness of symptoms may depend on the extent of your SCI.

Table 2 Bladder and kidney problems

Symptoms	What can be done
Bladder infection	
Urine with a strong or unusual odor Cloudy or reddish-brown urine An urge to urinate more often than usual Sudden urge to urinate Lower abdominal pain or cramping (may not be evident if you have a lack of sensation) Burning sensation when urinating (may not be evident if you have a lack of sensation) Low energy, feeling tired or mildly ill Incontinence Increase in general body spasticity (increased spasms in the body) Fever Autonomic hyperreflexia	Contact your health care provider so that a urine specimen can be collected to test for infection. Test results will also indicate which antibiotic is the best treatment, if you have an infection. To prevent bladder infections, follow your bladder management program.
Kidney infection	
High fever Severe headache Onset of midback pain (may not be evident if you have a lack of sensation) Increased bladder spasticity Chills Sudden stomach upset or nausea Autonomic hyperreflexia	Contact your health care provider immediately. If not treated quickly and appropriately, infections can damage the kidneys. Treatment with antibiotics may be necessary to prevent loss of kidney function. To prevent kidney infections, follow your bladder management program. Get prompt treatment for kidney infections.

(continued on next page)

Table 2 Continued

Symptoms	What can be done
Bladder stones	
Incontinence Increased bladder spasticity Repeated bladder infections Blood in urine Uncontrolled spasticity in arms or legs Autonomic hyperreflexia	Call your health care provider. Bladder stones often cause infection. The infection will persist until the stones are passed or removed. If the stones do not pass on their own, cystoscopy or lithotripsy may be needed. With cystoscopy, the stones are crushed and the pieces are removed through the urethra. Lithotripsy uses ultrasound waves to break up the stones so the pieces can pass on their own. To prevent bladder stones: Follow your bladder management program. Try to remain free of bladder and kidney infections.
Kidney stones	
If you have sensation, kidney stones can be very painful as they move through the ureters into the bladder. Watch for the following signs: Blood in urine Onset of midback pain Increased bladder or body spasticity Autonomic hyperreflexia	Call your health care provider. Bladder stones often cause infection. The infection will persist until the stones are passed or removed. If the stones do not pass on their own, cystoscopy or lithotripsy may be needed. With cystoscopy, the stones are crushed and the pieces are removed through the urethra. Lithotripsy uses ultrasound waves to break up the stones so the pieces can pass on their own. To prevent bladder stones: Follow your bladder management program. Try to remain free of bladder and kidney infections.

Autonomic hyperreflexia

Autonomic hyperreflexia (dysreflexia) is a potentially life-threatening rise in blood pressure which can occur in people with spinal cord injuries at or above a T6 injury. Bladder problems, such as those listed above, can cause autonomic hyperreflexia. See *Autonomic Hyperreflexia,* Chapter Four, for more information.

BOWEL MANAGEMENT

Introduction

Spinal cord injury (SCI) can affect the function of your bowel and may result in an inability to control bowel movements. This information discusses some changes in bowel function that may follow SCI and how to manage these changes.

Normal Bowel Function

When you swallow food, it moves through the digestive system; down the esophagus, into the stomach, to the small intestine and then into the large intestine (also called colon or bowel). As it moves, the food is broken down and the body absorbs nutrients and liquids. Stool (solid waste) is left in the bowel. The stool is moved into the rectum by wavelike movements of the bowel, called peristalsis. When the stool reaches the rectum, you have the urge to have a bowel movement (this urge may continue intermittently until you expel the stool). The anal sphincter of your rectum then relaxes and tightens allowing stool to be expelled in a controlled manner (Figure 11).

SCI-Related Bowel Changes

Normally, one can feel stool in the rectum and voluntarily contract the anal sphincter to hold stool and relax the anal sphincter to have

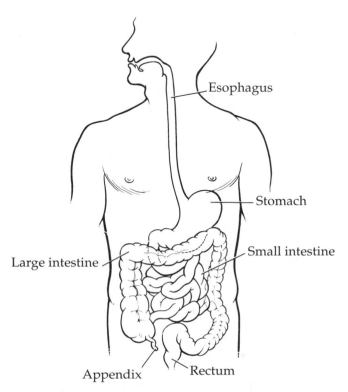

Figure 11. Digestive system.

a bowel movement. After SCI, bowel function and sensation may be altered. You may be unable to relax or tighten the anal sphincter. Therefore, your bowel movements may not be controlled. You may not know you have stool in the rectum or sense the urge to have a bowel movement. Spinal cord injury can also affect peristalsis. However, you can still control your bowel movements if you follow a regular bowel management program.

You may experience neurogenic bowel (loss of normal control of bowel function) from a problem such as SCI. Generally, there are two basic types of neurogenic bowel—upper motor neuron and lower motor neuron. The type of neurogenic bowel is based on the level of the SCI.

Upper motor neuron bowel (reflexic/spastic)
This condition typically results from SCI at the cervical (neck) or thoracic (chest) level. Messages between the colon and the brain are interrupted. Below the level of your injury, the spinal cord coordinates bowel reflexes. Your body still will have reflex peristalsis, although you may not feel the need to have a bowel movement. Stool may build up in your rectum, and trigger a reflex bowel movement (accident) without warning.

Between bowel movements, the anal sphincter remains closed. Your colon responds to digital stimulation and stimulant medications with reflex peristalsis, to push the stool out. The goals in managing an upper motor neuron bowel are to keep the stool soft yet formed, to empty the bowel on a routine basis (at least three times a week), and to prevent incontinence (accidents).

Lower motor neuron bowel (areflexic/flaccid)
This condition typically results from SCI at the lower end of the spinal cord—the lumbar (lower back) and sacral (pelvis) level or the nerve branches that go out to the bowel. This means that you have reduced peristalsis and decreased tone and voluntary control of your anal sphincter. Lower motor neuron bowel may not respond to digital stimulation. However, manual removal of stool may be necessary. The goals in management are to keep the stool well formed, to empty the rectum daily, and to prevent incontinence.

Bowel Management

To prevent bowel problems, it is important to follow a regular bowel management program. This program includes a proper diet, adequate fluid intake, physical activity, and emptying your bowel on a regular schedule. Also included may be the use of medications such as bulk-forming agents, stool softeners, stimulants, osmotic laxatives, suppositories and enemas.

Diet

A diet high in fiber helps regulate stool consistency and softness. It also promotes regular bowel movements by stimulating peristalsis. You should have at least eight servings of fiber-containing foods each day, which is equal to 20 to 30 grams of fiber per day.

Major sources of fiber are:
- Whole grain breads and cereals
- Fruits and vegetables
- Legumes, beans, lentils and nuts

Certain foods or beverages may upset your bowel program by either increasing or decreasing bowel activity. Through experience, you will learn which foods affect your bowel function. See Table 3 for a general list of foods that may harden or soften your stool.

Table 3 Dietary effects on bowel management

Food group	Foods that harden stool	Foods that soften stool
Carbohydrates	White rice, enriched noodles. Any food made with white flour such as white bread, crackers, cereals, pancakes, sweet breads, bagels, and biscuits.	100% whole grain breads and 100% whole grain cereals, red wine
Fruits and Vegetables	Fruit juices without pulp, bananas, apples without skin, potatoes without skin	All vegetables, all fruits with skin except bananas
Dairy	Milk, yogurt made without fruit, cheese, cottage cheese	Yogurt with seeds or fruit, buttermilk
Protein	Any meat, fish, poultry, or peanut butter without nuts	Seeds, nuts, lentils, chunky peanut butter, processed meats, dried beans
Fats	None	All
Desserts and Sweets	Any without fruit or seeds	Black licorice, any made with fruit or seeds, chocolate
Other		Artificial sweeteners such as sorbitol, xylitol, mannitol, and fructose, caffeine, cola, tea, spicy foods

Fluids

Fluids help keep your stool soft. The general recommendation is to drink at least 1.8 liters per day (8 to 10, eight-ounce glasses). However, since a change in how much fluid you drink may affect your bladder management program, discuss your recommended fluid intake with a member of your health care team.

Physical activity

Regular physical activity is important because it promotes regular bowel movements. See *Fitness*, Chapter Seven, for more information.

Medications

Medications can play an important role in effective bowel management. Your health care team will determine medications needed for your bowel program.

Some common medications that are used with bowel management are:

Bulk-forming agents: Often called fiber supplements, help regulate the consistency of stool by absorbing and holding water. This increases stool bulk and stimulates peristalsis. It is important to drink sufficient fluid while using bulk-forming agents. The combination of fiber and fluid gives your stool a moderately soft and formed consistency.
Bulk-forming agents include:
• Psyllium (Metamucil™)
• Methylcellulose (Citracil™)
• Calcium polycarbophil (Fibercon™)

Stool softeners: Draw water into the stool to help keep it soft and prevent constipation. Occasionally, your stool may become too soft. The result may be an accidental bowel movement. If this happens, reduce the dosage or stop taking the stool softener. Start again when your stool is well formed.
Stool softeners include:
• Ducusate sodium (Colace™)
• Mineral oil

Stimulants: Make the colon contract more forcefully. They increase the wavelike action, to move stool through the bowel faster. If taken by mouth, these medications should be taken 6 to 8 hours before expected or planned bowel care.

Stimulants include:
- Senna (Senokot™)
- Bisacodyl (Dulcolax™)
- Cascara
- Castor oil

Osmotic laxatives: Increase stool bulk by pulling water into the colon. They also stimulate bowel activity. It is important to drink a sufficient amount of fluids with these medications.
Osmotic laxatives include:
- Magnesium hydroxide (Milk of Magnesia™)
- Lactulose
- Magnesium citrate (Citrate of Magnesia™)
- Sodium biphosphate (Fleet Enema™)
- Polyethylene glycol (MiraLax™)

Suppositories/mini-enemas: Medications inserted into your rectum. They help to stimulate peristalsis or lubricate bowel contents.
Suppositories/mini-enemas include:
- Dulcolax™
- Enmeez™

Enemas: Large-volume enemas, overstimulate the bowel and decrease its natural tone and movement. Enemas should be used only as directed by your health care provider.
Enemas include:
- Fleet™
- Tap water enema

Bowel Problems

Following SCI, you may experience one or more of the bowel management problems outlined in Table 4.

Table 4 Bowel problems

Problem	Signs	Causes	What to do
Constipation (Hard, infrequent stools)	Hard or marble-like stool. No bowel movement for several days. Hard or swollen lower abdomen.	Not having enough fluid or fiber in your diet. Lack of activity. Not staying on your bowel care schedule. Lack of regularly scheduled bowel program.	Review your diet to make sure you are getting enough fiber and fluid. Repeat your bowel care the next day if you had a small, hard stool, or no bowel movement.

Problem	Signs	Causes	What to do
Constipation (continued)	Lack of appetite pain or discomfort in your side or lower abdomen (depending on level of injury). Nausea and vomiting. Autonomic hyperreflexia.	Incomplete emptying of lower bowel. Medications (narcotics, iron). Psychological stress. Irritable bowel syndrome.	If you still have not had a bowel movement after repeating bowel care, take one tablespoon of Milk of Magnesia™ 8 to 12 hours before your scheduled bowel care. Repeat your bowel care at the scheduled time. If you still have poor results, contact your health care provider. Increase activity/range of motion. Add stool softener.
Impaction (Partial or complete blockage in intestine by stool)	Many of the same signs as constipation. Loose or watery stools. Low-grade temperature. Autonomic hyperreflexia.	Liquid is being pushed or is leaking around hard stool that is blocking the rectum. (Impaction may result from constipation.) Same as constipation.	If stool is blocking your rectum, remove it gently with a gloved, lubricated finger. Be alert to the potential for autonomic hyperreflexia (dysreflexia). See *Autonomic Hyperreflexia*, Chapter Four, for more information. If you suspect impaction and cannot feel stool blocking your rectum, seek medical attention immediately.
Rectal bleeding (Bright red blood on your stool, toilet paper, or glove)	Painful bowel movements depending on the level of your injury. Bright red blood on stool or under- garments. Swollen skin tags at anal opening.	Passing hard stools over a long period of time. Digital stimulation or removing stool with your finger. Hemorrhoids. Rectal fissures (cracks or breaks in the skin). Straining from both bowel movement and bladder emptying.	Soften stool. Gentle digital stimulation without trauma. If this continues for 2 to 3 bowel programs, contact your health care provider. Hemorrhoids usually improve in two or three weeks with some changes in your bowel care routine.

Problem	Signs	Causes	What to do
Diarrhea (Loose stool)	Abnormally frequent, loose, watery stools. Unplanned bowel movements (accidents). Irritable Bowel Syndrome.	Dietary changes (for example, eating spicy or fatty foods). Illness (flu or intestinal infection). Medications (may be the side effect of antibiotics, or overuse of laxatives or stool softeners). Possible impaction. Caffeine (coffee, tea, or cola). Psychological stress.	Check your rectum for stool. If any is present, remove it gently. Stop taking stool softeners, suppositories or laxatives until diarrhea clears up. If you take a bulk-forming agent, check with your health care provider before continuing to use it. Be sure to continue all other medications unless your health care provider tells you otherwise. Review your diet, medications and bowel care program to find the cause of your diarrhea. Keep your rectal and genital area clean and dry. Moisture and stool can cause skin irritation and possibly a bladder infection. If diarrhea continues for three days, call your health care provider.
Incontinence (Unplanned bowel movement)	Unscheduled or accidental bowel movements.	Stools are too soft and oozing out. Eating more food than before. Overuse of laxatives. Eating too many stimulant foods. Not following your bowel care program.	Continue your regularly scheduled time for bowel care. You may need to do bowel care more frequently. Review your diet, fluid intake, medications and bowel care routine and try to find the cause. If the stool was loose or watery, stop taking your stool softener

Problem	Signs	Causes	What to do
Incontinence (continued)		Rectum not completely empty with bowel care.	until the stool returns to its normal consistency. If incontinence continues despite your efforts to correct the problem, call your health care provider.
Excessive gas (Abnormal amount of air in the intestinal tract)	Bloating of the abdomen. Frequent passing of gas that may or may not result in a bowel accident. Abdominal pain.	Consumption of gas-forming foods. Constipation. Swallowing air while eating or drinking (drinking through a straw). Artificial sweeteners (mannitol, sorbitol). Carbonated beverages.	Eat food slowly, chew with mouth closed. Establish a bowel care program. Certain foods may cause gas (especially fruits such as apples, honeydew, cantaloupe, watermelon or vegetables such as beans, broccoli, brussel sprouts, cabbage, cauliflower, onion, also carbonated beverages. Trial periods of omitting food one at a time can help determine the cause.

Bowel Care

The purpose of your bowel care program is to stimulate the lower bowel (colon) and rectum to empty their contents at a convenient time. Therefore, it is important to establish a set (consistent) time for bowel care. The best time is usually about 30 minutes after a meal. This lets you take advantage of your body's normal reflexes. You may need to insert a suppository and/or do digital stimulation (outlined below).

You will need the following supplies:
- Clean gloves (consider latex-free gloves, since you may have allergies)
- Water-based lubricant (such as K-Y™ jelly)
- A suppository (prescribed by your health care provider or an over-the-counter from your drugstore) or mini-enema

- Bed protector (such as Chux™), if bowel care is done lying side-ways in bed
- A commode if you cannot use the toilet

Procedure

- Place a bed protector under your buttocks and lie on your left side, knees slightly bent, your right leg crossed over the left, if you are doing bowel care in bed. If you cannot lie on your left side, ask a member of your health care team about other positions.
- Wearing gloves, generously lubricate your finger and insert it gently into your rectum. If stool is in your rectum, remove it carefully using your finger.
- Insert the suppository, pointed end first, high into the rectum and against the rectal wall. Place the suppository as high up into your rectum as you can reach with your finger. The suppository will not work if you insert it into stool, so you must remove any stool in the rectum as directed above.
- If you use a mini-enema, twist the top of the plastic applicator off and lubricate the tip. While lying on your left side in bed, squeeze contents of the mini-enema into your rectum and discard the plastic applicator.
- After you insert the suppository or mini-enema, wait 10 to 20 minutes for it to work.
- If you can transfer from the bed, it is best to complete the bowel care on a commode or toilet. Using the commode/toilet will feel more natural when having a bowel movement and gravity will also assist.
- Next, do digital stimulation by inserting a gloved, lubricated finger into your rectum. Do not insert your finger any further than 1 to 1½ inches into your rectum. Gently rotate your finger in a circular motion for about 10 to 45 seconds, touching rectal wall. This will stimulate peristalsis. Do digital stimulation every 5 to 10 minutes until you have results. Repeat the digital stimulation after you have had results to make sure you have completely emptied your rectum. Slight bleeding may occur as a result of digital stimulation, especially if you have hemorrhoids. It is important to do digital stimulation gently and to keep your fingernails short.
- Clean the rectal and genital area after the bowel movement.
- Generally, you will finish bowel care within one or two hours. This time frame varies from person to person. With experience, you will learn how much time you need.
- If you are unable to have a bowel movement using a suppository or digital stimulation, repeat this process again the next

day. If you still do not have results, please review suggestions under "constipation" in Table 7.

- Check your rectum for stool. If any is present, gently remove it.

Note:
Autonomic hyperreflexia (dysreflexia) may occur during bowel care and rectal digital stimulation. Finding comfortable position- ing during bowel care or utilizing anesthetic ointment on the anal area prior to the start of bowel care may prevent or relieve signs or symptoms of autonomic hyperreflexia. See *Autonomic Hyperreflexia*, Chapter Four, for more information.

Surgery

Colostomy or ileostomy are surgical procedures done to create an opening (stoma) on the abdomen where stool can be pushed out into an attached disposable bag. The surgery is called colostomy or ileostomy depending on where the opening is made in the intesti- nal tract. Goals of this surgery are to improve your quality of life by making you more independent in bowel care, reducing bowel care time and effort, and/or preventing bowel accidents. Deciding on surgery is a serious matter and must be done for the right reasons. Talk to members of your health care team to decide if surgery is the right choice.

3 Dealing with Skin, Muscle, and Bone Function

SKIN CARE

A body organ is a unique structure with a specific function essential to your well-being. Your skin is the largest and most visible organ. Your skin's functions are vital for the following reasons:

- To provide a protective barrier against infection and injury
- To feel sensations such as touch, temperature and pressure
- To help control body temperature

After a spinal cord injury/dysfunction, your ability to move or feel parts of your body changes. The degree of change depends upon the extent of your injuries. These changes can leave your skin prone to problems that result from lack of sensation, movement, injury or poor hygiene.

The purpose of this chapter is to help you understand how to protect and care for your skin after SCI. This includes identifying potential skin problems and the actions to take if you discover a problem.

Caring For Your Skin

The following care guidelines may help prevent skin problems.

- *Keep your skin clean and dry:* Shower or bathe your entire body once a day. Dry your skin thoroughly. Use warm water, soap, a clean washcloth and towel to wash and dry your genital and rectal area in the morning and evening. If you become soiled with urine or stool, wash and dry again.

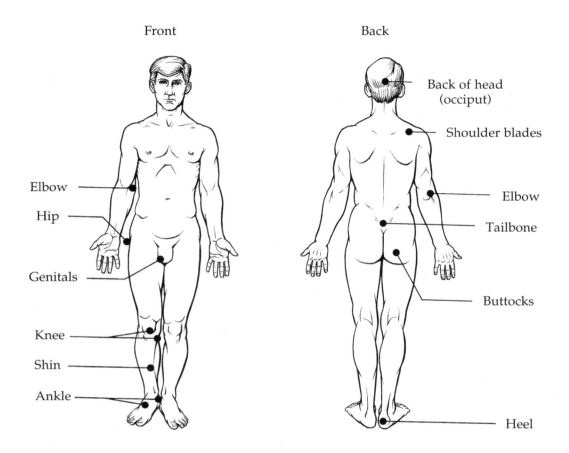

Front

Back

Elbow

Hip

Genitals

Knee

Shin

Ankle

Back of head
(occiput)

Shoulder blades

Elbow

Tailbone

Buttocks

Heel

Figure 1. Areas to check.

- *Examine your skin at least twice a day:* Check your skin for changes in color, temperature, swelling, unnatural wrinkles or rashes. Use a long-handled mirror to help you see all parts of your body. Check your skin when you awaken and before you go to bed at night, and after transferring from your wheelchair to your bed. Familiarize yourself with your skin's normal appearance so you will notice skin changes.
- The most critical areas to check are the back of your head, your shoulder blades, elbows, hips, tailbone, genitals, buttocks, knees, shins, ankles and heels (Figure 1). Your skin may be reddened or pink in these areas immediately after you change positions. If the area remains red after 15 minutes, you need to stay off that area until it is no longer red or pink.

Pressure Ulcers

A pressure ulcer is an injury to tissues caused by a long period of constant pressure or a brief period of intense pressure, which decreases the amount of blood flow to areas of your skin. Without enough blood flow, these affected areas become starved for nutrients and oxygen.

After a few hours of constant pressure or a brief period of intense pressure, the affected skin and tissues may become red. This change in skin color may be the only symptom that a pressure ulcer is developing, until an open sore appears a few days or weeks later. If steps are taken to relieve pressure on the reddened area, it is possible to prevent a pressure ulcer from developing. Pressure ulcers can also be prevented by carefully avoiding key factors that cause them, such as those listed below.

Causes

Key factors that may decrease blood flow to tissues and cause pressure ulcers include:

- *Pressure:* May result from factors such as sitting or lying on hard surfaces, thick seams in clothing, tight-fitting clothing or shoes, wrinkled clothing or sheets, or a wheelchair that does not fit your body properly.
- *Friction:* Changing your body's position is the key to preventing pressure ulcers. However, the friction of sliding from side to side or from one surface to another can damage your skin and cause pressure ulcers to develop.
- *Shear:* When your skin moves in one direction and the underlying bone moves in another, shear can result. Shearing can stretch, tear or bend tiny blood vessels and damage your skin, especially in areas where skin is thin and fragile. For example, sliding down in bed or a chair frequently may cause shearing over the tailbone. Lying in bed with the head elevated puts you at high risk for shearing over the tailbone and should be avoided if possible.
- *Moisture:* Perspiration, urine or other moisture can soften skin and make it more fragile. Moisture may also give bacteria a place to grow and cause an infection.
- *Temperature:* Heat and humidity can cause increased accumulation of moisture from perspiration, contributing to pressure ulcers.

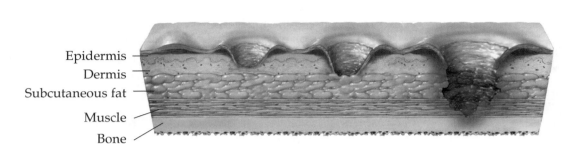

Stage 1   Stage 2   Stage 3   Stage 4

Epidermis
Dermis
Subcutaneous fat
Muscle
Bone

Figure 2. Stages of pressure ulcers.

Progression

Pressure ulcers can begin in deep muscle layers and progress outward to the skin, or they may develop on the surface of the skin and progress inward. Pressure ulcers are classified by stages, based on type and severity of tissue damage (Figure 2).

The stages of pressure ulcers are:

- *Stage I:* A pressure ulcer begins as a red area on the skin. This reddened area may or may not feel hard and/or hot. If you have black skin, the area may appear shiny instead of red. At this stage, the progression of an ulcer is reversible. Remove pressure from the area until the skin returns to normal color.
- *Stage II:* A blister or open sore, which involves the skin layers epidermis and dermis.
- *Stage III:* The ulcer may be small at the surface of the skin, but larger in deeper tissues. This damage extends to or through the subcutaneous fat.
- *Stage IV:* Damage through all layers of tissue occurs, with exposed muscle, tendon or bone.
- *Suspected deep tissue injury:* This may be a purple or maroon area of discolored skin, or a blood-filled blister due to damage of underlying soft tissue. This change in color may be preceded by the area being firm or boggy to the touch and/or warmer or cooler compared to other parts of your skin.
- *Unstageable:* Typically has damage through all tissue layers. However, the surface of the ulcer is covered with thick, leathery, dead tissue.

Complications

Pressure ulcers can lead to bone infections called osteomyelitis. When this occurs, you may experience pus-like drainage from the ulcer as well as pain and inflammation in the area surrounding the ulcer. Many persons also have a fever with osteomyelitis.

In order to heal osteomyelitis, you may need to be on prolonged bed rest for up to several months. This can alter functional, social, recreational and vocational activities. Bed rest can also lead to muscle weakness, impaired ability to transfer from your wheelchair, and mood difficulties.

Some ulcers may require surgical intervention for healing. The remaining scar tissue is very fragile and at high risk for re-injury. Pressure ulcers may cause increased spasticity or autonomic hyper-reflexia.

Prevention

You can prevent pressure sores by:
- Maintaining correct posture when sitting. Use positioning straps and supports as recommended.
- Using a properly fitted seat cushion and wheelchair. Place a pressure-reducing surface on your bed and/or chair as recommended by your therapist. These surfaces can include foam, air or gel.
- Do not adjust your chair, particularly the footplate height, without monitoring your skin closely for redness. Your therapist can assist with the appropriate modifications.
- Relieve pressure on your skin every 15 minutes when sitting in your wheelchair. Some methods to relieve pressure include:
  — Leaning from side to side.
  — Shifting your position in the wheelchair.
  — Placing your feet flat on the wheelchair footrest and bending forward as if to put your chest on your thighs.
  — Doing wheelchair push-ups from your elbows or hands as recommended by your therapist.
  — Use the capability of an electric wheelchair to shift positions.
- When lying in bed, turn every two or three hours.
- Before using sport or racing wheelchairs, talk with a health care team member or therapist. These wheelchairs are designed with less padding. A unique frame is designed with a tighter seat angle and may not provide sufficient protection.
- When traveling by car or public transportation, use your wheelchair seat cushion or travel cushion to help relieve pressure. You need to be aware that the inflation of an air-filled cushion changes in pressurized airplanes. Take frequent breaks and change positions often while in your seat.

- When selecting clothing (including underclothes), choose clothes that fit well. Clothing that is too tight may bind and place pressure on your skin. Clothing that is too loose may bunch up or form a ridge that also places pressure on your skin. Smooth clothes under you when you sit or lie down.
- Eat a healthy diet and make sure to drink enough fluids.
- Maintain weight within 10 percent of your ideal weight. See *Nutrition*, Chapter Seven, for more information.
- Wear shoes during the day to protect feet and toes.
- Watch for and control swelling so there is not increased pressure when wearing shoes or braces.
- Ask your therapist about pressure mapping to assess your pressure distribution when sitting in your chair or cushion.
- Maintain your wheelchair and seat cushion as recommended, particularly if you use an air-filled cushion.
- With SCI, as your skin ages you will need to alter how you relieve pressure. Review with your therapist strategies and additional techniques to protect your skin over time.

It is important that you do not:
- Use a rubber air ring or any kind of doughnut (inflatable circular chair cushion). They can increase pressure and block the blood flow to the skin inside the ring.
- Wear clothing with heavy seams, nylon underwear or tight clothing.
- Put items in your pants pockets or on the seat of your wheelchair.
- Use tobacco, because it impairs circulation, which is necessary for healthy skin.

Other Skin Problems

Edema

Edema (swelling) may occur in your paralyzed limbs if they remain in one position for several hours, or if your footrests are incorrectly positioned too low. Swelling can also result from poor blood circulation in your paralyzed limbs and you may notice puffiness, particularly in your hands and feet. Swollen skin is more easily injured.

Prevention

Raise your arms to shoulder level and rest them on pillows or wedge supports intermittently during the day. Raise your legs to hip level and rest them on another surface, keeping pressure off your heels.

Elevation during the night and intermittently (at least every two hours) during the day can help prevent edema.

Bruising

Bruising may occur when small blood vessels just under the skin surface are broken and blood leaks into the surrounding tissue and you may notice red-or purple-colored skin. Bumping yourself when transferring to or from your wheelchair can cause bruising.

Prevention

When transferring, do not "drag" your buttocks across your wheelchair or other surfaces. Gently lift and lower your body. Wear clothing or place a towel under your buttocks if you use a transfer board, unless your therapist has shown you another method of transferring. The wheelchair seat with cushion should be about the same height as the surface to which you are transferring, to allow for an easier, safer transfer. Move your legs carefully to prevent bruising your heels and ankles.

Ingrown toenails

Toenails can grow into the surrounding skin, causing inflammation, pain and infection. The most common causes of ingrown toenails are improper clipping or wearing shoes or socks that are too tight. Red and inflamed skin around a toenail is a sign of an ingrown toenail.

Prevention

Toenails should be cut straight across, even with the end of the toe (Figure 3). Rough edges of toenails should be filed smooth. Avoid wearing tight-fitting shoes and socks, which can increase the possibility of ingrown toenails.

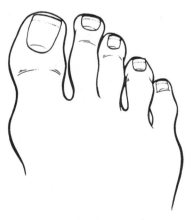

Figure 3. Toenails cut straight across.

Skin rash

Moist skin in areas not exposed to air, drug allergies and skin infections are major causes of rashes. A rash may also result from prolonged contact with urine, feces or sweat. Red, irritated skin may indicate a skin rash.

Prevention

Keep your skin clean and dry. Avoid direct contact with substances that cause rashes, such as cleaning products.

Burns

Exposure to excessive heat can damage your skin. Because parts of your body may not feel heat, you can burn yourself without knowing it. Hot liquids, bath water, heating pads, cigarettes, radiators and sunlight may cause burns. Red, blistered, white or charred skin may result from burns.

Prevention

When bathing or showering, always test the water temperature with a thermometer to be sure the water does not exceed 96 degrees Fahrenheit (35.5 degrees Celsius). To protect your skin, set your water heater thermostat at a lower temperature to avoid water that might be too hot to touch. Smoking is discouraged. However, if you smoke, do not let ashes or matches fall on your clothing. Never hold an ashtray in your lap or smoke in bed.

When cooking, do not lift pots with boiling contents from the stove or put hot liquids where they might spill on you. Keep handles turned inward on the stove. Pour hot liquids, such as coffee, away from your body, not over your lap. Do not hold hot foods, such as a hot coffee mug or pizza from a hot oven, in your lap.

When using a heater in your car or house, check the distance between the heat source and your feet and legs often. Keep at least six feet between you and space heaters, hot pipes, radiators, wood-burning stoves or fireplaces. In your car, leave at least six inches between heat vents and your feet and legs.

When in the sun, use a lotion with an SPF (sun protection factor) of 30 or greater on exposed skin and limit time in the sun to brief periods. Pay particular attention to the tops of your feet if they are exposed to the sun.

Frostbite

Just as burns may occur because your body may not feel heat, frostbite may occur because parts of your body cannot feel cold. Frostbite occurs when skin areas are overexposed to cold air or cold objects (such as a car air conditioner, frozen food, or ice packs). Red, white, gray or blistered areas on your skin may result from frostbite.

Prevention

When outdoors in cold weather, dress for the conditions. Take breaks from the cold often and check exposed skin for signs of frostbite. When using an air conditioner in your car, leave at least six inches between the cool air vents and your legs and feet. Do not place or hold cold or frozen items such as containers with frozen food or ice cubes in your lap.

Genital Hygiene

Good genital hygiene is especially important after a spinal cord injury to prevent skin irritation and to control the growth of bacteria that could cause a urinary tract infection. Keep your body clean and dry, especially areas where you perspire. This is particularly important in your genital and rectal areas where bacteria can spread quickly.

Use warm water, soap and a clean washcloth and towel to wash your genital and rectal area once in the morning and again in the evening. If you become wet during the day, wash and dry again.

Special skin care considerations for men

Each time you wash, start with the penis and pubic hair. If you are not circumcised, pull your foreskin back and wash the head of your penis completely. Return foreskin over the head of your penis after cleansing. Next wash your scrotum, thighs, rectal area and buttocks. Rinse thoroughly and dry completely.

If you wear an external "condom catheter," wash and dry your entire genital and rectal area as described above and check your skin every time you put on a condom. Change the condom daily, even if it is not leaking. Expose your penis to the air as long as possible between condom changes. If possible, use a urinal at night instead of wearing a condom.

As you are putting on a condom (if you are not circumcised), pull the foreskin toward the head of your penis. This prevents a constricting or "tourniquet" effect that could impede blood circulation, causing swelling and skin breakdown. Roll the condom down until the entire penis is covered. If you have an erection while putting on a condom, be sure to check the condom later to make sure it is on securely. For specific directions on condom application, follow the instructions from the manufacturer.

Check the condom often to see that it is draining properly. Be sure it is not twisted and that you used the correct size. Check for correct fit by making certain that you can easily put on and remove the condom. Check the condom again for proper fit about 15 minutes after you put it on. If you see signs of leakage, swelling or skin color changes in the head of your penis, remove the condom immediately. Wait for the swelling or color to return to normal before applying another or different size condom.

Special skin considerations for women

When cleansing your genital area, always wash from the front toward the back. Next, wash your thighs, rectal area and buttocks. Rinse thoroughly and dry completely.

Although SCI does not have a direct effect on your menstrual cycle, your menstrual periods may stop for awhile immediately following your injury. Within a few months to as long as a year, your menstrual cycle, or "period," should resume. If it does not, talk with your health care provider. If your periods occurred at regular intervals before your injury, they may continue at regular intervals.

After your SCI, you may need to consider how you will handle your menstrual flow. If you use sanitary napkins, clean your genital and rectal area each time you change a napkin. Check your skin often where it comes in contact with the pad, especially the inner thighs and buttocks. If you use tampons, you will need the ability to transfer yourself and to insert and remove tampons with your hands. Depending upon your hand use and transfer abilities, tampons may be difficult to use.

Identifying Skin Problems

The information in Table 1 on the next page may help you identify skin problems and guide you in resolving them. Treating skin problems promptly can help prevent further complications. If a condition persists or becomes severe, call your health care provider immediately.

MUSCLE, BONE AND JOINT CHANGES

Following spinal cord injury, you may experience changes in your muscles, bones, and joints. This section explains some of these changes and possible complications.

Table 1 Skin problems

Problem	Signs of a problem	What you can do
Pressure ulcer See Figure 2 for more information.	Redness on an area of skin indicates pressure has cut off the blood supply. Skin loses its normal pink color and appears white or gray or a blister forms, indicating the skin has become damaged or tissue has died. An open sore may form in the damaged tissue, leading to a serious infection.	Remove the source of pressure. Skin color should return to normal in 30 minutes.
Swelling (edema)	Puffy hands and/or feet	While sitting in a chair or lying in bed, raise your hands or feet on pillows for several hours. Wear compression garments.
Burn	Red skin	Remove the source of heat. Apply cold (not ice) water compresses with a clean towel or place your skin under cold running water (cover area with a cloth).
	Blistered skin	Apply cold (not ice) water compresses with a clean towel or cloth. Elevate the blistered area.
	White or charred skin	Apply cold (not ice) water compresses with a clean cloth or towel.
Frostbite	Red area	Warm affected skin by adding warm coverings (without placing pressure on affected part), or re-warm affected area quickly in warm (not hot) 96 degrees Fahrenheit water.
	White- or gray-skin	Use a thermometer to make sure the water is not hotter than 96 degrees Fahrenheit. Do not rub with snow or ice.
	Blisters	Try to re-warm as described above.
Rash	Red, irritated area	Cleanse and dry the of skin area and leave it open to the air.
Bruise	Red- or purple-colored skin	Protect and prevent from further injury; watch for healing.
Ingrown toenail	Red, inflamed skin around a toenail	Talk to a member of your health care team.

Muscle Tone

Muscles are made up of elastic like fibers that relax and contract to produce movement. The amount of tension or resistance to movement in muscles is defined as muscle tone. Muscles may be slightly tense or partially contracted to hold your body in a natural position.

Muscle tone after SCI

Your brain and spinal cord control muscle tone and balance. After SCI, the tone in your muscles may be changed. Muscles may develop too much tone and become spastic (rigid and contracted), or lose too much tone and become flaccid (limp and soft).

Spastic Muscles

You are more likely to have spastic rather than flaccid muscles after SCI at or above a T10 level. Spastic muscles may be tight when you are sitting or resting in bed, may be loose most of the time with intermittent jerking or cramps, or may cramp when you try to walk or move a muscle. Some people have "clonus" or involuntary repetitive jumping of the leg when the foot is moved or calf is stretched. These symptoms may or may not be problematic. Having spastic muscles is not always bad and in fact may have many advantages.

Advantages and disadvantages of spasticity
Some advantages of spasticity include:
* Warning sign of problems that you can't feel, such as pain, urinary tract infections (UTI) and pressure ulcers.
* Helps maintain muscle tone, bulk and physique.
* Promotes circulation and possibly prevents blood clots.
* Provides tone for transfers or walking.

Some disadvantages of spasticity include:
* Interferes with activities of daily living, including dressing, bathing and transfers.
* Friction or shearing of the skin.
* Joint contractures: Tightness of the tissue around joints and in muscles, causing limitations in joint movements.
* Pain.
* Awakening at night.

Treatment of spastic muscles

Many treatments help control spastic muscles and prevent joint contractures. The two primary treatments are exercise and medication.

Exercise

A consistent program of stretching, positioning, weight bearing for legs, and task activities for arms and hands can modify spasticity. A therapist can teach you the correct techniques, which include tension and timing of the stretches. Other exercises may include range of motion, alternating limb movements such as bicycling, locomotor (walking) training, and strengthening exercises. When exercising, it is important to stretch frequently throughout the day, make sure you are positioned correctly, and put weight on your joints as instructed by your therapist.

Medication

If stretching exercises are not effective, medication may help decrease spasticity. Your health care provider may first prescribe baclofen (Lioresal™) or tizanidine (Zanaflex™). Side effects of these medications can include drowsiness and weakness. If baclofen or tizanidine is ineffective, other medications such as diazepam (Valium™) and dantrolene (Dantrium™) may be added or substituted. Side effects must be carefully monitored to help determine appropriate dosages. Periodic tests of liver function may be needed when taking these medications. Researchers continue to develop other drugs to treat spastic muscles. Talk to your health care provider to determine if medication is appropriate for you.

Other treatment methods

Other spasticity treatments may help, depending on your goals. Options include, but are not limited to:

- *Functional Electrical Stimulation (FES):* Electrical stimulation to provide activity to affected nerves or muscles.
- *Intrathecal drug pump:* Medication is placed directly into the thecal sac which surrounds the spinal cord, through a drug pump implanted under the skin. This stops the nerve from sending signals to the muscles and decreases spasticity. The pump must be refilled every 1 to 6 months, depending on pump size and your dose.
- *Intramuscular neurolysis:* Certain muscles are injected with botulism toxin (Botox™). This procedure provides temporary relief of spasticity, allowing motion and strengthening of muscle groups as part of a therapy program and can be repeated every three months.
- *Motor point blocks:* Similar to intramuscular neurolysis, a phenol solution is used to stop communication between nerve and muscle. This procedure can only be performed in one or two areas of your body at a time and may need to be repeated every 6 to 12 months.

Neurological and orthopedic surgery may be an option of last resort. Discuss this opion with our health care provider.

Flaccid muscles

Flaccidity (having flaccid muscles) may develop shortly after a T10 or lower SCI and may or may not persist. Flaccidity allows limbs to be easily moved and thus eases positioning and dressing. Flaccid muscles tend to become thinner and smaller, known as atrophy. Flaccidity can increase your risk of developing pressure sores and blood clots (deep venous thrombosis or pulmonary embolus).

Managing flaccid muscles

Techniques to manage flaccid muscles and protect your joints include:
- Proper positioning with pillows and frequent changes in body position.
- Proper lifting and transferring techniques.
- Use of splints or braces to support your extremities, maintain functional positions, and avoid injuries.
- Daily exercises as instructed by your therapist.

Bone Changes

The bones of your skeletal system perform many vital functions, including:
- Provide shape and form to your body
- Protect your vital organs
- Produce blood cells
- Store salts and minerals

The bones of your spinal column contain the nerves of your back. Disease or injury can affect any part of your spinal column or nerves. Skeletal changes and complications can result from an injury or disease of the spinal cord. Changes and complications can also occur as you age, because of:
- Immobility or lack of movement
- Positioning
- Posture
- Aging
- Overuse

Bone Conditions Related to SCI

Hypercalcemia

Hypercalcemia (excess calcium) is a complication that may occur one to twelve weeks after SCI. Typically this condition is short-lasting, but without corrective treatment, can persist up to one year.

Adolescent males with a complete cervical injury who become de-hydrated and are immobilized for a time are at greatest risk for developing this condition immediately following SCI. However, everyone with SCI is at some risk.

Hypercalcemia results in decreased bone formation and an in-creased rate of calcium absorption in the body. Flu like symptoms such as loss of appetite, nausea, vomiting, headache, fatigue, stom-ach pains, increased thirst and behavioral changes may accompany this condition. Fortunately, this rarely occurs.

Diagnosis and treatment
Hypercalcemia is confirmed by checking calcium levels in the blood and urine. Treatment includes lowering calcium levels through in-creased fluid intake, medications (such as pamidronate disodium or etidronate disodium) and regular physical exercise beginning as soon as possible following injury.

Prevention
Increasing daily fluid intake to at least eight, 8-ounce glasses (or the amount recommended by your health care provider) and daily exercise may help prevent hypercalcemia.

Heterotopic ossification (HO)

Heterotopic ossification (HO) occurs in 20 percent to 30 percent of people with spinal cord injury. HO is most common in people who have spinal cord injuries above the waist. It affects the joints below the level of injury, resulting in abnormal deposits of new bone formation around joints, in the muscle, and between muscle fibers (Figure 4). The hip, knee, elbow and shoulder joints are most commonly affected.

Symptoms of this condition include joint or extremity redness and swelling, increased skin temperature of the affected area, decreased range of motion, discomfort or pain, increased spasticity and auto-nomic hyperreflexia.

Another complication is complete ankylosis (stiffening and fusing together of the joints) or loss of movement in joints due to bone deposits. This complication may require surgery to restore range of motion, but in most cases, HO should not pose a problem for those with a spinal cord injury.

Diagnosis and treatment

HO is confirmed by X-rays, bone scans and blood tests. In most cases, regular exercise is the most important part of treatment. In

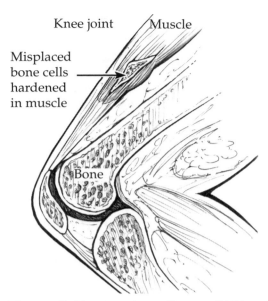

Knee joint   Muscle

Misplaced
bone cells
hardened
in muscle

Bone

Figure 4. Heterotopic ossification (HO) in the knee joint.

addition to increased activity and range of motion exercises, treatment includes medications such as indomethacin (Indocin™) or
disodium editronate diphoshonate (Didronel™), and radiation
therapy. Surgical removal is also a treatment option after the heterotopic bones have matured. Surgery is most successful if performed
after bone formation is complete, usually 12 to 18 months after SCI,
or the problem may recur.

Prevention

If you are at high risk for developing HO, you may receive preventive medication or radiation therapy before the condition develops.

Osteoporosis

Osteoporosis is a weakening of the bones that is caused by a loss of
important minerals such as calcium and phosphorus. Osteoporosis
causes the bones to become brittle and more likely to fracture easily. Most older adults, particularly postmenopausal women, have
some degree of bone loss as a natural result of aging. Regardless of
age, bone loss often occurs within six months after SCI.

Osteoporosis is often called the "silent disease" because bone loss
occurs without noticeable symptoms. You may not know that you
have osteoporosis until your bones become so weak that a sudden
movement or fall results in a fracture. Symptoms such as swelling
at the point of injury, abnormal alignment of the bone, or increased
muscle spasms may indicate a fracture. Hearing a "crack" is a sign

that a break may have occurred. Loss of muscle function results in decreased tension on the long bones of the legs, causing the bones to lose calcium and phosphorus, and become weak and brittle.

Diagnosis and treatment

Specialized tests can measure bone density to help detect osteoporosis before a fracture occurs. When conducted at intervals of a year or more, bone density testing can predict your risk of having fractures in the future, determine your rate of bone loss and monitor the effectiveness of treatment. Medications are available to treat osteoporosis. Fractures may require surgery in an effort to prevent complications such as improper healing.

Prevention

Engaging in daily exercise, particularly weight-bearing exercise, is important in helping to prevent osteoporosis. Work with your health care provider to create a program based on your needs and ability. Some people who have limited mobility can increase their bone strength by using a standing frame or table, standing wheelchair, parallel bars or braces. Tension on the bones while standing in these devices may slow bone loss. Refraining from alcohol, tobacco products and recreational drugs may also help prevent bone loss.

Abnormal spinal curvatures

Abnormal spinal curvature typically results from muscle weakness, paralysis, spasticity, bone destruction at the time of injury, or vertebral column changes following surgery (Figures 5–7). Types of abnormal curvatures of the spine include:

- *Kyphosis or hunchback:* Excessive upper back (thoracic) curve
- *Lordosis or swayback:* Increase in the curvature of the lower back (lumbar)
- *Scoliosis:* Lateral or sideways curvature ("S" shape) of the spine

Symptoms include neck and back pain, and poor posture. Serious spinal curvature can impair your ability to sit, maintain balance, breathe and participate in activities. Poor positioning and trunk support in your wheelchair may also result in spinal curvature, making it difficult to drive or propel the wheelchair. Severe deformities may impair heart and lung function, which can lead to trouble breathing or pneumonia.

Diagnosis and treatment

Diagnosis of abnormal spinal curvatures is made by physical examination and spinal X-ray. Treatment of spinal curvatures may include wheelchair modifications, bracing and surgery.

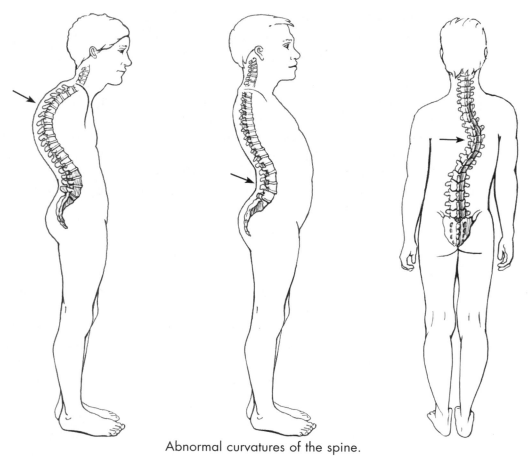

Abnormal curvatures of the spine.

Figure 5. Kyphosis.   **Figure 6.** Lordosis.   **Figure 7.** Scoliosis.

Prevention

Abnormal spinal curvatures can often be prevented through proper seating and positioning (Figure 8). Yearly evaluations are important for early detection.

Overuse Conditions

People with injury or disease of the spinal cord often develop upper extremity joint problems. Each day your upper extremity joints must repeatedly do tasks that they were not designed to do, such as propelling a manual wheelchair, transferring from one surface to another, or walking with crutches and walkers. As a result, upper extremity pain can occur during rehabilitation or years later. Common conditions caused by overuse include carpal tunnel syndrome and shoulder pain. People who have incomplete injuries may also

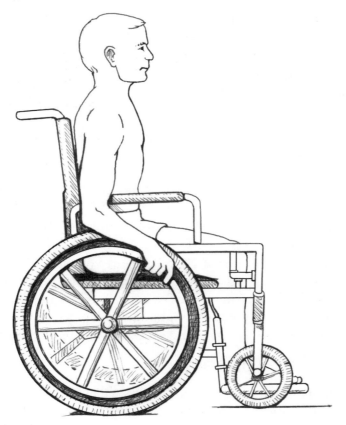

Figure 8. Correct posture while seated in a wheelchair.

experience conditions in their lower extremities such as hip bursitis, ankle instability or strain, and overuse of knee ligaments. Strengthening, fitness and assistive technology are important interventions to decrease overuse injuries.

Overuse can affect any joint, but with care and strengthening, many problems can be prevented. Assistive technology and mobility devices can help. Talk to your therapist for more information about these prevention techniques and those listed below.

Shoulder pain

Shoulder pain can occur anytime as a result of immobility, positioning, transferring and overuse. With SCI, shoulder pain can result from the trauma that caused your injury. Signs and symptoms include pain when you lift your arm out to the side of your body, a dull ache, sharp pinch, radiating pain, increased muscle tone and poor posture.

Diagnosis and treatment
Diagnosis is made through physical examination. The goal of treatment is to relieve pain and inflammation, and allow exercise and movement. Treatments include pain-free, range of motion exercise, pain and anti-inflammatory medications, cold and heat therapy, protection from further injury (correct positioning, safe transferring, avoiding overuse), rest and perhaps surgery.

Prevention
Prevent shoulder pain by:
- Carefully positioning your arms and shoulders when you lie or sit.
- Avoiding transfers that stress or pull on the joints of your arms and shoulders.
- Avoiding positions that could injure your shoulders and tendons.
- Avoiding overuse. Heed pain symptoms and discontinue positions or movements that cause or increase pain.
- Consulting your occupational and physical therapists about how to prevent pain and scheduling regular evaluations.

Carpal tunnel syndrome

Carpal tunnel syndrome occurs when a nerve entering your hand is trapped between tendons in your wrist. As you bend and flex your wrist, pain, burning, numbness and tingling may occur in your wrist, hand and arm. These sensations often occur at night when your wrist is at rest.

Diagnosis and treatment
Diagnosis of carpal tunnel syndrome is made through physical examination and electromyography (EMG). Treatment may include adjusting assistive equipment, modifying activities to reduce wrist stress, or wrist splints, cortisone injections, oral anti-inflammatory medications, and perhaps surgery.

Prevention
Avoid repetitive motion of the wrist, especially flexion (bending the wrist down). If you use a wheelchair, using push gloves or adding pegs to your chair wheels, or using power assist wheels may help reduce the strain on your wrists. Using a power chair temporarily or permanently also may help protect your wrists from a repetitive motion injury. If you use crutches or a cane, a padded or custom-molded hand grip may help reduce pressure on the carpal tunnel. Wearing a wrist splint may relieve symptoms during the night.

4 Managing Circulation and Body Regulation

CIRCULATORY CHANGES

Following spinal cord injury, you may experience changes to your circulatory system, which includes your heart, arteries, veins and capillaries. The purpose of this chapter is to explain the anatomy and normal function of the circulatory system, as well as changes and potential problems that you may experience following your injury.

Normal Anatomy and Function

The heart pumps blood through several types of blood vessels. The blood carries nutrients from food and oxygen from your lungs to every part of your body. Arteries carry fresh, oxygen-rich blood away from the heart and lungs to tissues throughout the body (Figure 1). Veins return blood containing waste products, such as carbon dioxide, back from tissues throughout the body to the heart and lungs. In the lungs, the carbon dioxide is exchanged for a fresh supply of oxygen.

Circulatory System Changes and Problems

Spinal cord injury disturbs the regulation of blood pressure, heart rate, and how blood moves from the body back to the heart. Some circulatory system changes and problems you may experience following SCI are:

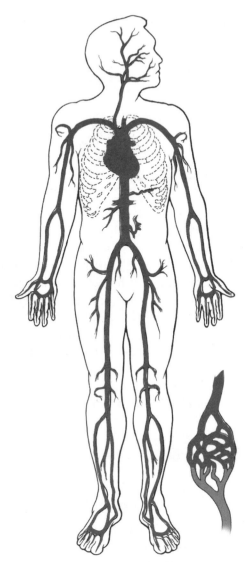

Figure 1. Arteries in the body.

Spinal shock

Depending on your level of injury, you may experience spinal shock following SCI. This condition occurs immediately following your injury and may last from a few days to a few weeks. It is accompanied by flaccid (soft, limp, without muscle tone) paralysis below the level of injury.

Symptoms of spinal shock include:
- *Hypotension:* Low blood pressure

- *Bradycardia:* Heart rate slower than normal range
- *Hypothermia:* Body temperature below normal range

The higher the level of injury, the more symptoms you may experience.

Prevention
This condition cannot be prevented, as it occurs naturally with your injury.

Orthostatic hypotension

Orthostatic hypotension is a sudden, severe drop in your blood pressure when you stand after sitting, or sit up after lying down. This drop in blood pressure may make you feel dizzy or faint. Normally, when a person stands (or sits after lying down), the effects of gravity cause blood pressure to drop slightly because blood is being pulled into the legs. Your body normally compensates for the increased blood flow to the legs by constricting (narrowing) blood vessels and increasing heart rate. This response involves your autonomic nervous system, which controls body functions such as blood pressure and heart rate.

After SCI, the autonomic nervous system does not work properly. Your resting blood pressure may decrease because blood vessels cannot constrict as efficiently as they did before your injury. Therefore, when you sit up or stand, blood pools in your abdominal cavity and legs.

A sudden drop in blood pressure can decrease the amount of blood to your brain, perhaps causing:
- Light-headedness
- Fainting
- Blurring, graying or loss of vision, tunnel vision
- Fatigue
- Feelings of unsteadiness
- Confusion or difficulty thinking

Prevention
To help prevent orthostatic hypotension:
- Change positions slowly. For example, raise the head of your bed while resting intermittently before transferring to your wheelchair, or sit at the edge of the bed for a moment before standing.
- Wear elastic stockings with or without elastic bandages on top. Some people require compression stockings, prescribed by their health care provider, for long-term management.

- Wear an abdominal binder.
- Increase your fluid intake.
- Elevate your legs.
- Avoid hot showers.

If symptoms continue despite these measures, consult your health care provider. You may need medication to raise your blood pressure. Medication options may include midodrine, fludrocortisone and others. Talk to your health care provider to determine if medication is appropriate.

Edema

Edema (swelling) may occur in paralyzed limbs if they remain in one position for more than several hours, or if footrests are positioned incorrectly. Swelling can result from poor blood circulation in paralyzed limbs.

Symptoms of edema may particularly affect the hands and feet and include:
- Puffiness
- Pain or stiffness

Prevention
Tips for preventing edema include:
- Move or have someone help you move the swollen limb. Movement can help decrease swelling by returning fluid in the limbs back to the heart.
- Raise your arms to shoulder level, rest them on pillows, or wedge supports under them throughout the day.
- Raise your legs to hip level, rest them on another surface, keeping pressure off your heels.
- Elevate your limbs during the night.
- Use compression (elastic) stockings, sleeves or wraps.

Compare your extremities. Swelling in only one, or more swelling in one than the other, may be a sign of a deep venous thrombosis.

Deep venous thrombosis and pulmonary embolus

Arteries carry blood away from the heart to circulate throughout the body, and veins carry blood back to the heart. Gravity and muscle contractions help move the blood through the arteries and veins. When blood moves slowly or pools in the veins, a blood clot may form, perhaps resulting in deep venous thrombosis (DVT) or pulmonary embolus.

Blood clots

Blood clots are more likely to form in the veins, especially leg veins, where blood may pool. People with SCI who have paraplegia (paralyzed legs) are at risk of forming blood clots in the leg veins. People who have quadriplegia (paralyzed arms and legs) may be at risk for developing clots in their arms and legs. An additional risk factor in developing blood clots is a family history of tendency to form blood clots. Therefore, to assist in determining your risk and plan of care, inform your health care provider of any family history of blood clots.

A blood clot that stays in one place is called a thrombus. A clot that breaks free and travels to another part of the body, such as the lungs or brain, is an embolus.

Deep venous thrombosis

Deep venous thrombosis is a blood clot that forms in a vein and typically occurs in the arms or legs. The risk of DVT is highest within the first three months after your injury. Because health and risk factors vary, talk to your health care provider about how often you and your caregiver should check your arms and legs for symptoms of DVT.

Symptoms of DVT may include:
- Increased swelling in only one arm or leg.
- Redness of the skin.
- Increased spasticity: An increase in the deep tendon reflexes, which may cause them to feel tight and rigid. This symptom also may cause an exaggerated knee-jerk reflex.
- Increased warmth: One arm or leg that is warm to the touch compared to the other.
- Low-grade fever at night: Temperature above 101.5 degrees Fahrenheit or 38.5 degrees Celsius for two days.
- **Autonomic hyperreflexia (dysreflexia):** A potentially life-threatening increase in blood pressure which can occur with SCI at or above a T6 injury level. See *Autonomic Hyperreflexia*, later in this chapter, for more information.

If you have signs or symptoms of DVT, go to your health care provider or emergency department immediately. Meanwhile, remove any leg bag straps and constrictive clothing except support stockings. Your health care provider or emergency room physician may request special tests, such as an ultrasound or computed tomography (CT), scan to determine if you have DVT.

Pulmonary embolus

An embolus is the most dangerous type of blood clot. It is a clot that breaks off, floats away in the bloodstream and lodges elsewhere. A pulmonary embolus is a clot that has traveled to the lung and blocked blood flow.

Symptoms of pulmonary embolus may include:
- Feeling of breathlessness.
- Sudden chest pain, which may worsen when inhaling.
- Coughing up bright red secretions (saliva or phlegm).
- Fast heartbeat (palpitations).
- Shallow or more rapid breathing.

If you have symptoms of pulmonary embolus, immediately call 911. This condition is extremely dangerous and, if not treated, can lead to death.

Prevention

Because very slow blood flow is a main reason blood clots form in veins, improving blood flow is one way to reduce the risk of deep venous thrombosis and pulmonary embolus. To improve blood flow:
- Elevate (raise) your legs for 15 to 20 minutes, 2 to 3 times a day.
- Perform range-of-motion exercises.
- Wear support stockings or elastic wraps. Talk to your health care provider about which is more appropriate.
- Check your arms and legs daily for swelling or redness, which may indicate DVT.
- Stay well hydrated by drinking plenty of fluids.
- Avoid nicotine.
- Avoid the use of constricting items or garments such as straps of leg bags, garters, elastic stockings with tight bands and knee socks. These may decrease blood flow.
- Take anticoagulant (blood thinning) medication as prescribed by your health care provider. Anticoagulant medications may include low molecular weight heparin, Fragmin™, or Lovenox™. Three months after injury, these medications may no longer be necessary, as the risk of DVT declines. Since a risk of bleeding is associated with anticoagulation medication, the use of this medication requires very close medical supervision. Blood tests may be done as often as every day until the level of the medication in your blood is appropriate.

Treatment

If your health care provider diagnoses you with DVT or pulmonary embolus, treatment will start immediately and may consist of bed rest, medication and perhaps hospitalization. Leg elevation and special compression stockings are also potential treatments for DVT or pulmonary embolus.

Anticoagulation. Your health care provider may decide that you should start or continue anticoagulation medication to prevent more blood clots. The most common anticoagulation medications used to treat DVT and pulmonary embolus are heparin and warfarin (Coumadin™). Heparin is most commonly given first, either by injection or intravenously (IV). Intravenous medication involves placing a catheter into a vein. Warfarin is usually given by mouth and is used for treatment at home. Warfarin may be continued for 3 to 6 months, or indefinitely, as determined by your health care provider.

You need to know the details about all of your medications. Tell your health care provider about any medications, including over-the-counter, that you take. Medications such as aspirin or antibiotics can change the effect of anticoagulants. Because of potential risk factors, ask your health care provider about how to use anticoagulation medications safely at home and include your questions or concerns.

Bed rest and leg elevation. During the diagnosis and early treatment phases of DVT you may need to remain in bed with your affected leg or arm constantly elevated (raised). This position helps decrease swelling caused by the blood clot. Your health care provider will determine when bed rest can be discontinued and activity resumed.

Compression devices. Support stockings and elastic wraps (compression devices) may help reduce the pooling of blood in your legs by promoting blood flow. They may also help reduce swelling.

Prevention is the best treatment for DVT and pulmonary embolus. Because blood clots may recur, continued preventive care is important. Check your legs and arms daily for signs of a blood clot (swelling, redness, increased spasticity and warmth). If you notice any sign, promptly go to your health care provider or emergency department.

Cardiovascular disease

Cardiovascular disease is the leading cause of death among men and women. However, in persons with SCI, cardiovascular disease appears to occur earlier than might be expected under normal circumstances. Physical inactivity and weight gain decrease muscle and lean body mass, increasing the percentage of body fat and the risk for cardiovascular disease after SCI. Due to changes in activity level, chest wall sensation (inability to feel your chest area) and pain perception, cardiac disease symptoms may present as referred pain (pain that is felt somewhere other than where it originated) and autonomic hyperreflexia. Therefore, various screenings such as blood tests, X-rays and exercise testing may be needed.

Blood cholesterol tests can help identify your risk for cardiovascular disease. This test measures total cholesterol, levels of low-density lipoprotein (LDL or "bad") cholesterol, high-density lipoprotein (HDL or "good") cholesterol and blood fats called triglycerides. Cholesterol is a fatlike substance produced by the liver. It also enters your body when you eat food that contains animal fat. High cholesterol increases the risk of clogged arteries. If an artery leading to the brain becomes clogged, stroke can result. If an artery in your heart becomes clogged, heart attack can result. Poor diet and lack of physical activity result in decreased HDL cholesterol levels and elevated LDL cholesterol levels. HDL cholesterol is thought to help protect against cardiovascular disease.

Prevention
Prevention of cardiovascular disease includes:
- Regular physical activity
- Do not smoke
- Maintain an ideal weight by losing weight, if necessary
- Dietary factors
  — Reduce saturated fats, trans fats and cholesterol in your diet
    - Saturated fats are found mainly in animal products, including whole milk, cheese, butter, beef, pork, lamb, as well as palm oil, coconut oil, cocoa butter and hydrogenated oils.
    - Trans fats should be avoided. These fats are found in baked goods, processed foods, some margarines, shortening and some forms of peanut butter.
  — Moderate consumption of monosaturated fats, with no more than 30 percent of calories coming from fat. Monosaturated fats help lower blood cholesterol levels if eaten in limited amounts. They can be found in olive, peanut and canola oil.
  — Limit consumption of sodium. Sodium attracts and holds water in the body and excess fluid retention can put added stress on the heart and blood vessels to pump the extra fluid. The recommendation by the American Heart Association is 2,000 to 3,000 mg per day. Foods to limit include pre-

packaged items, fast food, canned soups and vegetables, deli meats, cheese, snack foods and condiments (soy sauce, ketchup, salad dressing).

— Increase fiber intake to help lower cholesterol. Soluble fiber is found in citrus fruits, strawberries, apples, legumes, oatmeal and oat bran, or as a supplement. Insoluble fiber stimulates the GI tract and is found in foods such as vegetables, wheat bran and whole wheat grain breads. The recommended amount to consume is 10 grams to 25 grams per day of soluble fiber and at least 25 grams to 30 grams of total fiber per day.

— Increase consumption of sterols or stanols, which have been found to reduce LDL cholesterol levels. Examples of products that contain sterols or stanols are Benecol™ and Take Control™. Recommended levels are 2 grams per day, every day. Typically, results can be seen after two weeks of correct use.

— Consume omega 3 fatty acids, which help prevent cardiovascular disease. The American Heart Association recommends 1 gram of omega 3 fatty acids per day. Good sources are fish and fish oils. At least two servings of fish are recommended per week.

— Limit alcohol intake to 1 to 2 servings per day, which may reduce cardiovascular disease risk.

— Bake, broil, steam or grill foods. Avoid frying to reduce calories and fat.

BODY TEMPERATURE CONTROL

Spinal cord injury can affect your body's ability to control its temperature. This section discusses some changes in body temperature control that may follow SCI and how to manage them.

Temperature Control

The body normally maintains its temperature within a narrow range. This regulation mechanism is complex; sensors in the skin respond to temperature changes in the environment and send messages to control centers in the body. Following SCI, this sensing and regulation system may not function normally. Your body may not be able to generate heat by shivering, or cool itself by perspiring. Without this control, your body tends to take on a temperature similar to the environment. For example, if a person is indoors, their body takes on the indoor temperature. Persons with a higher level of spinal cord injury are more prone to these changes.

Temperature extremes

Prolonged exposure to cold temperatures can cause your body temperature to fall below normal. The result can be loss of consciousness and possibly death. Prolonged exposure to heat and humidity can cause your body temperature to rise to dangerous levels. The result can be dehydration, convulsions, kidney problems and possibly death.

Besides temperature extremes, other factors such as alcohol intake and fever may also alter your temperature control. Do not drink alcohol outside in the cold, because it dilates your blood vessels, resulting in body heat loss. Too much alcohol can also lessen your awareness of your environment and impair your judgment.

Infection may cause a fever that could result in a very high body temperature. Therefore, you may need fewer clothes and covers, so that heat can escape from your body. If you are ill with a fever, talk to your health care provider about your body temperature and your symptoms.

Preventing Problems

Knowing the temperature of the environment and planning ahead are the best ways to prevent body temperature problems. The following suggestions may help:
- Wear the right clothing for the weather conditions.
- Be aware of and ready to respond to changes in weather.
- Ask your health care provider if you should avoid direct sunlight and stay in the shade.
- Arrange for reliable transportation that has functioning heating and cooling systems.
- Check your home to make sure heating and cooling systems are working properly.

If you have a problem controlling your body temperature, contact your health care provider.

AUTONOMIC HYPERREFLEXIA

A spinal cord injury can affect your body's circulatory system. These effects may cause circulatory problems, such as autonomic hyperreflexia (also called autonomic dysreflexia), which is a serious rise in blood pressure.

Autonomic Hyperreflexia

Autonomic hyperreflexia is a medical condition that can occur in people who have SCI at or above the sixth thoracic (T6) level. It is the body's response to a painful or noxious (harmful) stimulus, such as an overfull bladder or bowel. Before your SCI, such stimulus would have caused pain or discomfort. However, with SCI, you lose feeling below the level of the injury. Therefore, the same stimulus goes unnoticed and may trigger autonomic hyperreflexia.

Autonomic hyperreflexia occurs when:
- Painful or noxious stimuli cause your body to send messages to your spinal cord. You don't feel the stimuli since the message cannot travel up the injured spinal cord to your brain.
- The painful or noxious stimuli cause blood vessels in your legs and abdomen to get smaller (constrict). The result is increased blood pressure, headache, goose bumps and pale skin below the level of injury.
- Other nerves send messages about your blood pressure increase to your brain. Your body then tries to decrease your blood pressure by:
  — Slowing down your heart rate
  — Dilating (expanding) blood vessels in your neck, face and upper chest. This causes a flushed, red or blotchy appearance above the level of injury.
  — Sending messages to blood vessels below the level of injury to dilate. However, this message is blocked by your spinal cord injury. Therefore, your blood vessels stay small, blood pressure stays high and may even continue to rise, which can cause serious medical conditions such as seizures, renal failure, or stroke.

Autonomic hyperreflexia is a medical emergency. Therefore, it is important to be aware of its triggers, symptoms, treatment and prevention.

Triggers

Autonomic hyperreflexia is most commonly brought on by a problem in the urinary tract or bowel (such as overfilling), since you may not be able to feel when your bladder or bowel is full. Additional key bladder or bowel triggers include:

- A plugged, indwelling catheter
- Urinary tract infection
- Kidney or bladder stones
- A stool impaction/constipation
- Bowel care

Other triggers of autonomic hyperreflexia may include:

- Pressure ulcer
- Prolonged pressure on skin (tight trousers, socks, or braces)
- Ingrown toenails
- Lower extremity stretching
- Blood clots in leg
- Childbirth
- Cystoscopy or other surgical procedures
- Sexual activity
- Bone fractures
- Conditions such as appendicitis or inflammation in the abdomen

Symptoms

Common symptoms include:

- Headache
- Sweating
- Flushing and reddening of skin above the level of injury
- Goose bumps below the level of injury
- Shortness of breath
- Feeling of unexplained anxiety, for example, "something is wrong"
- Pale skin below the level of injury

The most common signs of autonomic hyperreflexia include sudden high blood pressure and slow heart rate. Your blood pressure may rise 20-40 mm Hg (top number) above your normal level. For example, many persons with spinal cord injury at or above the T6 level have a blood pressure between 90 and 110 mm Hg systolic. If your normal systolic blood pressure is 110 and it suddenly increases to 130-140, you might be experiencing autonomic hyperreflexia. Inform your health care provider of your normal blood pressure numbers.

Autonomic hyperreflexia symptoms are usually mild but require prompt treatment. Occasionally, they may be severe or long-lasting, perhaps damaging your heart, blood vessels or brain. Stroke or heart attack can occur if autonomic hyperreflexia is not treated.

Treatment

The most important treatment for autonomic hyperreflexia is to remove or relieve its cause. If autonomic hyperreflexia develops:

- Return to bed and raise your head with pillows or raise the head of your bed if possible.
- Loosen any tight clothing, especially an abdominal binder. Check your skin for areas of redness or pressure.
- Feel your abdomen for distention or swelling.
- If you have an indwelling catheter, check that it is not plugged or clamped.
- If you do not have an indwelling catheter, you should be catheterized to relieve pressure in your bladder.
- With your finger, check your rectum for stool, using a numbing gel such as xylocaine as a lubricant. If you need bowel care, again use a numbing agent. If symptoms recur, stop, wait until they decrease, and then finish your bowel care.

Medication

Medications are available to treat autonomic hyperreflexia. Medications may be used when:

- Your blood pressure is dangerously high and needs to be reduced quickly.
- Autonomic hyperreflexia recurs so frequently that medication is needed constantly.

Talk to your health care provider to determine if medication to treat autonomic hyperreflexia is an option for you.

An informational pocket card on autonomic hyperreflexia can be carried with you at all times. This pocket card is available at www.pva. org and will be useful to individuals attending to you in emergent situations. Talk to your health care provider for more information.

Prevention

You can help prevent autonomic hyperreflexia by being aware of what causes the condition to occur and avoiding those triggers. Practice good bladder, bowel and skin care. See *Bladder Management* and *Bowel Management,* Chapter Two, and *Skin Care,* Chapter Three, for more information.

III

Sexuality and Fertility

5 Sexual Health

Sexual health is a state of physical, emotional, mental and social well-being in relation to sexuality. Sexual health requires a positive and respectful approach toward sexuality and sexual relationships. For many people, a spinal cord injury or disease affects sexual health. Specifically, the physical changes following SCI may affect your sexual function, as well as your self-image as a sexual being.

This chapter discusses sexuality and fertility following SCI. Although this information focuses on a heterosexual perspective, self-sex (masturbation) and same sex behavior are alternative choices.

Sexuality, Sex Drive and Sexual Activity

Sexuality involves the expression of your sex drive through sexual activities. However, sexuality is more than sexual behavior. It involves how you convey your gender (male or female). For example, the way you dress, the friends you choose and places you go, and how you articulate your talents and feelings. Every person is a sexual being, and the need for sexual expression is rarely lost following SCI. Your own view of yourself as a sexual being will influence how others view you. How you convey your sexuality is determined by factors present before you became disabled.

Your sex drive is a primary force, like hunger and thirst. Your hormones and nervous system regulate this drive. Illness, pain and anxiety may reduce sex drive. A disability by itself, however, does not affect sex drive.

Sexual activities are how you satisfy your sex drive. Sexual activities include hugging, stimulation of genital areas and erogenous zones (ears, neck, lips), and sexual intercourse. If you find previous sexual activities difficult to perform now that you have a disability, you may want to consider trying those activities in a modified way, or try new sexual activities.

Intimacy

Intimacy means being very familiar or closely associated with an-other person. It typically develops through spending time with another person, sharing innermost thoughts, feelings and desires. If you are married, or in an ongoing relationship, you may be fac-ing the re-establishment of your intimate and sexual relationship. Good communication forms the basis of a satisfactory sexual rela-tionship. Talking about your disability can reduce the impact it has on intimacy. Ask about your partner's sexual likes and dislikes, and respond with yours.

After SCI, many people wonder if sexual activity will cause pain or other discomfort. Encourage your partner to question you and the rehabilitation team members about changes to expect. Eliminating unnecessary fears can make resumption of intimacy and sexual ac-tivity easier.

How SCI affects sexual function differs for each person. You may want to spend time exploring your body. Knowing what feels good will help you tell your partner what he or she can do to make your sexual activities pleasurable. Experiment with ways to increase sex-ual pleasure by trying different positions and activities.

For those not in an intimate relationship prior to becoming dis-abled, dating may be a concern. Again, communication is key. Your partner must understand the nature and scope of your injury early in the relationship.

You can help by asking your partner:
- What would you like to know about my disability?
- Does my condition bother you?
- Are you concerned about other people's reactions to my dis-ability?
- Would you like to know how I feel about having a disability?

Be open and honest about your physical limitations. As a result, discussions later about more difficult topics, such as bladder man-agement and altered sexual function, become easier. Effective com-munication skills take practice but are worth the effort.

Re-establishing intimacy and sexual activity

If your SCI seems to impair your intimate relationship, consider:

- *Start slowly:* Effort, patience and persistence are necessary to maintain what is good in a relationship and remedy what is not. Give yourself and your partner time to get reacquainted and to make changes. Before focusing on improving your sexual relationship, spend time just talking to and being with your partner.
- *Stay positive:* Problems also can be opportunities. In your efforts to become more intimate, you may discover something new about your partner. Working together, you may find your relationship becomes stronger than it was before your injury.
- *Express your thoughts and feelings:* Intimacy begins with honest communication. Create an environment where you both feel comfortable sharing thoughts and feelings. Talk with your partner about how you feel, what you miss and what you want or need from the relationship. If you don't feel comfortable discussing certain topics, consider writing about them in a journal or a letter (even one you do not plan to share).
- *Listen:* Learning how your partner feels is important. Ask your partner to share his or her wants and needs, and express how your injury has affected him or her. Try to listen objectively, without feeling guilty or becoming defensive.
- *Find ways to rekindle romance:* Go out on a date, plan a picnic, send flowers or exchange personal gifts. Share ideas.
- *Be creative and willing to make changes:* Change could be as basic as purchasing a new mattress or bed so you don't have to sleep apart, or exploring different ways to express your sexuality.

Society and Sexuality

Society often treats people with disabilities as being sexless (asexual). If you accept society's narrow definition of who is "sexy," you may find that you do not fit this definition. Also, showing interest in sexuality may evoke negative reactions from others. They may be acting on their stereotypes of acceptable sexuality.

Try not to let negative stereotypes dictate how you act. Your appearance, body image and communication skills will greatly affect how others react to you. Communicating respect, self-acceptance and warmth may help others see you as a sexual person. Healthy sexuality and an active sex life can have a positive effect on all aspects of your life including health, self-esteem, relationships and productivity.

Anatomy

Reviewing human anatomy (Figures 1 and 2) is a step in under-standing how your sexual function may have changed as a result of your SCI.

Female

Bladder: Muscular organ that stores urine.

Cervix: Lower part of the uterus that has a small opening into the vagina.

Clitoris: Small, sensitive organ located in the labia, just above the vagina and urethra.

Fallopian tubes: Two tubes that carry an egg (ovum) from the ovaries to the uterus.

Labia: Folds of skin that cover the vagina, urethra and clitoris.

Ovaries: Glands that contain eggs, located on either side of the uter-us at the end of the fallopian tubes.

Urethra: Small tube that drains urine from the bladder.

Uterus: Pear-shaped organ at the top of the vagina which holds the developing baby during pregnancy. The lining of the uterus is shed every month (menstruation) if a woman is not pregnant and has not reached menopause.

Vagina: The canal that leads from outside the body to the uterus.

Male

Bladder: Muscular organ that stores urine.

Epididymis: A firm structure lying behind the testis that stores sperm.

Penis: External genital organ.

Prostate gland: Gland that produces fluid that mixes with sperm to make semen.

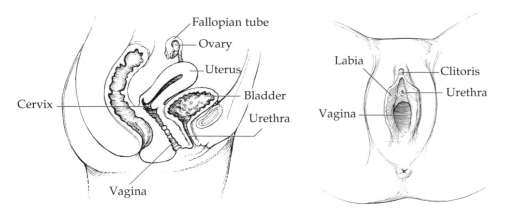

Figure 1. Female sexual anatomy.

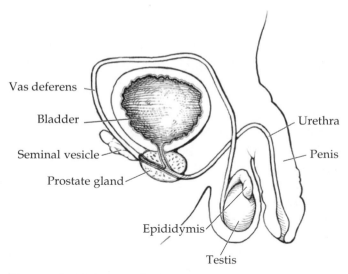

Figure 2. Male sexual anatomy.

Scrotum: Sac that holds the testes.
Seminal vesicle: Produces secretions that are added to the seminal fluid during ejaculation.
Testis: Gland that produces sperm.
Urethra: A small tube through which urine and semen travel from the bladder through the penis.
Vas deferens: A small tube that carries sperm from the epididymis to the urethra.

Sexual Response Cycle

Your body's response to sexual stimulation depends largely on your nervous system. The brain and spinal cord are important "relay stations" in the process of sexual arousal. Nerves extend from the spinal cord to your entire body, including the blood vessels, glands and skin in your genital area. These nerves send and receive messages through the spinal cord to and from your brain.

People may become sexually aroused when any senses are stimulated. Touch is the major source of stimulation, especially in the erogenous zones. These zones may include the ears, neck, lips, nipples or inner thighs. Although touch is an important part of sexual arousal, other senses have an active role. Smelling your favorite fragrance, listening to soft music or watching a sensual movie can increase your sexual arousal.

When a man is sexually aroused, nerves relay messages to blood vessels in the genital area, especially in the penis. When the blood vessels in the penis fill with blood, it becomes erect. When males have an orgasm, ejaculation usually occurs. Semen (sperm and seminal fluid) is discharged from the penis during ejaculation. The blood vessels in the penis empty following ejaculation, and the penis relaxes and becomes limp.

When a woman is sexually aroused, nerves send messages to blood vessels in the genital area. Blood flow increases, causing the labia to swell and the clitoris to become firm. Nerves also carry messages to glands in the vagina which produce lubrication and orgasm.

Sexual arousal occurs in two ways (Figure 3). One is psychogenic arousal (starting in the mind). This type of arousal is controlled by nerves at the T12 to L2 levels of the spinal cord. Psychogenic arousal can occur while thinking about sex, reading a romantic book or viewing sexually explicit pictures. As you become aroused, the brain sends messages to the spinal cord. The spinal cord forwards these messages to the genital area, resulting in physical sexual arousal.

The second type of arousal is reflexogenic (starting as a reflex). This type of arousal can result from touching the clitoris, labia, penis or other parts of the genital area. It is controlled by nerves at the S2 to

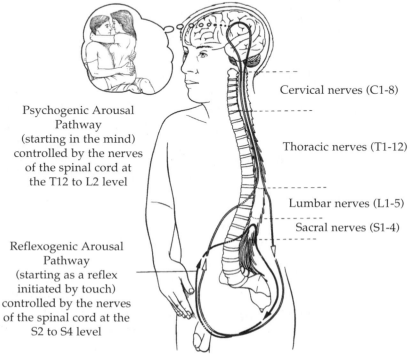

Psychogenic Arousal
Pathway
(starting in the mind)
controlled by the nerves
of the spinal cord at
the T12 to L2 level

Cervical nerves (C1-8)

Thoracic nerves (T1-12)

Lumbar nerves (L1-5)

Sacral nerves (S1-4)

Reflexogenic Arousal
Pathway
(starting as a reflex
initiated by touch)
controlled by the nerves
of the spinal cord at the
S2 to S4 level

Figure 3. Arousal pathway.

S4 levels of the spinal cord. These nerves first send messages from the skin being touched to the spinal cord. Then, the messages are relayed from the spinal cord back to blood vessels and glands in the genital area.

After your SCI, you may notice a change in sexual function. Men may notice changes in erection and ejaculation, whereas women may notice changes in lubrication. Your SCI may cause decreased or absent sensation and movement below the level of injury, but you may notice a heightened sensitivity in areas above the level of injury.

Male response cycle changes

Erection

Whether a man can have a psychogenic erection following SCI depends on the level and completeness of the injury. Men with low-level (below T10) incomplete injuries are more likely to have psychogenic erections. In contrast, men with complete injuries are less likely to have them.

Reflexogenic erections are usually possible unless your injury affects the nerves below the S1 level. An involuntary erection is possible due to a full bladder or stimulation to the genital area. You may have trouble keeping a reflexogenic erection.

If you cannot achieve or maintain an erection, and feel it is a major part of your sexual activity, here are some alternatives:

- *Vibromassage:* A vibrator provides intense stimulation to the penis. This stimulation sometimes causes an erection and/or ejaculation. It is important to learn how to use this method correctly to lessen the chance of side effects. Vibromassage can cause an increase in blood pressure, severe headache, or autonomic hyperreflexia (dysreflexia) in persons with injuries at T6 or above.
- *Penile implants:* Surgery that involves placing a flexible rod or an inflatable tube in your penis. These implants allow an erection, but do not restore sensation in the genital area. Penile implants cause significant risk of erosion of penile tissue and are used infrequently.
- *Oral medications (vasodialators):* Prescription medications (Viagra ™, sildenafil, tadalafil) that enhance the response to sexual stimulation by helping improve blood flow to the penis. When taken with vasodilators, some medications can cause dangerous drops in blood pressure. Talk with your health care provider or

pharmacist before you take Viagra™ or any medication that is used for sexual dysfunction.

- *Penile self-injection:* Medications injected directly into a vein on the penis also can produce an erection. Common medications are papaverine, phentolamine or prostaglandin. These medications increase the flow of blood to your penis and cause an erection. To use this technique, you or your partner must learn how to prepare the penis, draw up the medication into a syringe and inject it into the penis.

Priapism, a prolonged erection that occurs when blood does not drain from the penis, can occur with oral or injectable medication. Priapism can be painful and damage penile tissues, requiring medical attention if an erection lasts more than four hours. Therefore, you should consult with your health care provider if considering medication.

Talk to your health care provider about risks, benefits and methods to achieve and maintain an erection.

Ejaculation and orgasm

Ejaculation occurs when semen is forced out of the penis (Figure 4). Ejaculation is controlled by a combined and well-coordinated response of nerves and muscles. The nerves at the T12 to L2 levels send a message for the sperm to be forced into the urethra and for the bladder neck to close. The nerves at the S2 to S4 levels send a message to pelvic floor muscles to contract when the semen reaches the urethra and force the semen out of the penis.

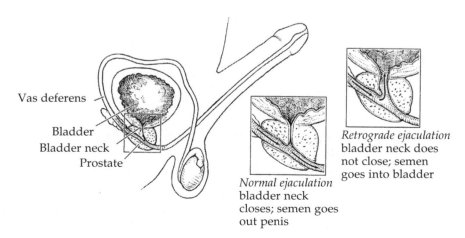

Vas deferens

Bladder
Bladder neck
Prostate

Normal ejaculation bladder neck closes; semen goes out penis

Retrograde ejaculation bladder neck does not close; semen goes into bladder

Figure 4. Ejaculation.

Some men with SCI may not be able to ejaculate. Retrograde ejaculations occur when semen flows backward into the bladder rather than out through the penis. Some men may have an orgasm without ejaculation or with a retrograde ejaculation. This is not a problem unless you are attempting to get your partner pregnant. Because of problems with ejaculation, most men with SCI must rely on alternative techniques such as vibromassage, to impregnate their partner.

Female response cycle changes

Lubrication

SCI can result in a lack of lubrication in women. A remedy is to use a water-soluble vaginal lubricant such as K-Y jelly™ or Astro Glide™. Water-soluble lubricants can help avoid vagina and labia skin breakdown. Do not use oil- or petroleum-based lubricants, such as Vaseline™. They do not dissolve in water and cannot be easily washed away. The buildup of lubricant can lead to infection. Also, oil-based lubricants may cause latex condoms to leak.

Orgasm

After SCI, you may lose the ability to have an orgasm. Orgasms vary in type and intensity among women. Many women with SCI who engage in sexual activity report that they experience orgasms. Those who do not experience orgasm can still have a pleasurable sexual experience. Some women with SCI describe a paraorgasm (a highly pleasurable feeling in parts of the skin and body that still have sensation). This does not depend on the motor or sensory function of your genital organs.

Preventing Sexually Transmitted Disease

Diseases such as gonorrhea, genital herpes or warts, human immunodeficiency virus (HIV) and chlamydia are sexually transmitted. They are passed from one person to another during intimate sexual contact. Such contact includes intercourse and oral or rectal contact with the sex organs. These diseases can affect persons with SCI just like anyone else.

Help prevent the spread of sexually transmitted diseases by taking these precautions:
- Talk to your partner about potential risk.
- Limit your number of sexual partners.
- Avoid sexual contact with a person who has a sexually transmitted disease or has a high risk for having such a disease.
- Use condoms.

Family Planning After SCI

Family planning is a conscious effort by couples to control the number and spacing of births, with natural and artificial birth control.

Preventing unplanned pregnancy

Birth control methods can be helpful for family planning. When deciding which birth control method to use, think about the following questions:
- How effective is this method?
- How safe is it?
- Am I comfortable with it from a health perspective and moral standpoint?
- Are there limitations to my using this method effectively?

There are various birth control options available. Talk to your health care provider about what form is appropriate for you, as well as the risks and benefits of each.

Barrier methods
These methods of contraception prevent sperm from reaching the egg. Barrier methods include a condom, diaphragm or cervical cap. When properly placed and used with a spermicide, they block sperm from entering the woman's cervix. Spermicides come in many forms and can be bought without a prescription. The diaphragm and cervical cap must be prescribed and fitted by a health care provider. These methods have fewer health risks than birth control pills or intrauterine devices (IUDs).

Correct placement of a condom, diaphragm or cervical cap requires good hand function. The diaphragm or cervical cap may become dislodged if you strain to empty your bladder. Therefore, you should check placement of the device and replace as necessary.

Natural family planning
Natural family planning involves monitoring changes in body temperature, vaginal mucus and the cervix to determine when a woman is fertile. Effectiveness depends on proper training and accurate record keeping. You will need good hand function to check your temperature, vaginal mucus and cervical changes. You must abstain from intercourse around the time of ovulation.

Hormonal medications
Birth control pills and time-released patches, rings and injections are examples of hormonal medications prescribed by health care

providers. These hormonal methods may not be recommended for women with SCI. They increase the risk of developing blood clots such as deep venous thrombosis (DVT). For more information on blood clots, see *Circulatory Changes* in Chapter Four.

Birth control pills contain hormones that prevent a woman's ovaries from producing a mature egg. Many types of birth control pills are available. If side effects occur, such as changes in weight, nausea, stomach cramps or breakthrough bleeding from one type, you may have better results with another. Birth control pills are highly effective if taken as directed.

Women can take hormones similar to those used in birth control pills in other time-released forms. Methods to deliver hormones include:
- A skin patch placed on your stomach or thigh, which you replace weekly.
- A ring that you insert in your vagina, leave in for three weeks and remove for one week.
- Injections given either once a month or once every three months by your health care provider.

Intrauterine device
An intrauterine device (IUD) is a small T-shaped device that is placed in a woman's uterus by a health care provider. It can stay in place for five years or longer. An IUD creates difficulty for an egg to implant in the wall of the uterus.

You must have good hand function and finger sensation to check placement of the IUD. Uterine or pelvic infections are risks with an IUD. If you have a loss of sensation below the waist, it may be difficult to tell if you have an infection.

Sterilization
Sterilization (surgically rendering a person incapable of reproducing) is a serious decision that should be made only after careful thought. Fertility can seldom be restored. If the possibility exists that you may still want to have children, you should choose another form of birth control.

The sterilization operation for women is called a tubal ligation. This procedure involves blocking the fallopian tubes (passages through which eggs travel to the uterus). After tubal ligation, a woman continues to produce an egg every month and have a period. However, because the fallopian tubes have been blocked, the egg and sperm cannot reach each other for fertilization to occur.

For men, the sterilization operation is called a vasectomy. It involves cutting and tying the vas deferens (the passage through which sperm leave the testicles). After a vasectomy, men continue to produce sperm, have erections and ejaculate. However, sperm cannot pass through the vas deferens. Without sperm, the woman's egg cannot be fertilized.

Both procedures are done on an outpatient basis. Recovery is usually rapid, within a few days. Ask your health care provider low long you must wait to have unprotected intercourse to avoid pregnancy after these procedures.

Pregnancy and child birth

After SCI, a woman's menstrual periods may not return to normal for a few months. During this time, you can become pregnant. Practicing birth control is important to avoid pregnancy. Your menstrual cycles can be managed the same way as before your injury. However, you will need to consider your hand function and ability to transfer when changing tampons or pads.

Spinal cord injury does not affect fertility in women. Most women with SCI can experience labor, have a normal delivery and breast-feed. While pregnant, you have increased risk of:

- *Urinary tract infections:* Maintaining a good bladder program is important. Your bladder management may need adjustment during pregnancy.
- *Constipation:* Maintain an effective bowel program. Altering your water or fiber intake may be necessary.
- *Pressure ulcers:* Weight gain and posture changes increase risk for pressure ulcers. You should check your skin more often. You may need to consult a physical or occupational therapist that specializes in wheelchair seating.
- *Spasticity:* You may need to wean off any spasticity medications while pregnant. You may also need to increase your stretching routine.
- *Autonomic hyperreflexia (dysreflexia):* For an injury above T6, pregnancy may increase the risk of autonomic hyperreflexia (dysreflexia), occurring secondary to bladder pressure, labor and delivery.

Your health care team can help you prevent or manage these issues. You and your health care provider should plan well in advance to prevent or manage possible problems during labor and delivery.

Male fertility

If you can ejaculate during sexual activity, you are fertile (unless you have had a vasectomy) and can impregnate a woman. To avoid a pregnancy, you must practice birth control.

Infertility in men is caused by the inability to ejaculate, low sperm count or poor sperm quality. Spontaneous erections following SCI may be irregular and difficult to predict. However, erections with ejaculation may be achieved through vibromassage or **electroejaculation**, which uses a rectal probe to electrically stimulate ejaculation. Electroejaculation must be done under a health care provider's supervision. In both methods, to induce pregnancy, semen is collected and artificially inserted into the women's uterus at a heightened time of fertility.

To determine if you are infertile, your health care provider can do a semen analysis. If low sperm count is a problem, more frequent ejaculations can improve sperm count.

Child rearing

Advanced planning and preparation will help prevent some problems you may experience while raising your child. You may need to modify your home to better manage parenting tasks. Seek different ways to assist with physical aspects of parenting. You may consider consulting an occupational or physical therapist for adaption of equipment. However, the most important aspect of successful parenting is effective communication skills between parents.

Managing Physical Changes and Medical Complications

A satisfying sex life is possible for people with SCI. However, you may need to confront issues such as positioning, spasticity, pain, autonomic hyperreflexia, involuntary bowel movements, bladder leaks and catheter management. If you wear a back brace such as a thoracic lumbar sacral orthosis (TLSO), or other types of braces, sexual activity may still be possible. Ask your health care provider for guidance.

Suggestions for you and your partner include:
- Discuss the potential issues listed above. Open communication can help prevent surprise or embarrassment.
- Communicate your needs to each other.

- Be open to sexual activities other than penile/vaginal intercourse.
- Experiment to find what is comfortable for both of you and what will reduce your fatigue.
- Ask your partner to help with your preparations, such as setting up supplies at bedside, positioning or other care needs.

Carefully explore your body for areas that give you pleasure. Do not overlook the parts that have reduced or no sensation. Decreased sensation in part of the body may trigger increased sensitivity just above the level of injury. Stroking or caressing this area can be especially pleasurable.

Positioning

You may find that the man-on-top sexual position will not work. The woman-on-top or side-to-side position may be more enjoyable. The following illustrations show various positions you may want to try. What you can do will depend on the level and completeness of your injury.

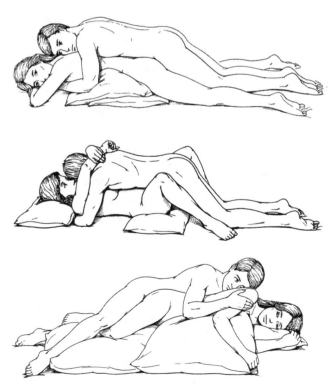

Figure 5. Sexual positions for women with SCI.

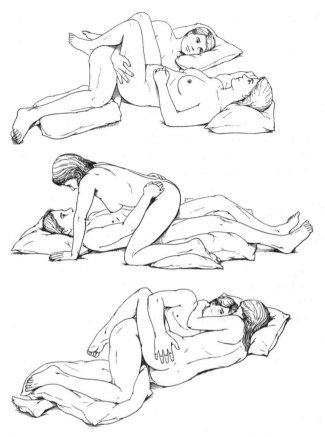

Figure 6. Sexual positions for men with SCI.

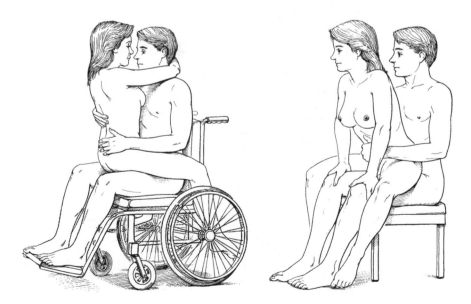

Figure 7. Sitting sexual positions.

Spasticity

Spasticity (increased muscle tone resulting in a tightening or short-ening of the muscles) can make positioning difficult. For position-ing problems, a warm bath before sexual activity may help. Relax-ation techniques, massage, gentle rocking, soft lighting and warm room temperature may also help relax and loosen your muscles. Experiment to find positions that decrease spasticity. Try stretching before sexual activity.

Pain

Pain may accompany sexual activity. For pain relief, try to deter-mine where and when the pain occurs. Experiment with different sexual positions to avoid pain. Use pillows for support and com-fort. If pain during sexual activity continues, seek the advice of your health care provider.

Autonomic hyperreflexia (dysreflexia)

If you have a spinal cord injury at or above the T6 level, a danger-ous rise in blood pressure, known as autonomic hyperreflexia (dys-reflexia), may occur during sexual activity.

To avoid autonomic hyperreflexia (dysreflexia) during sex:
- Empty your bladder before having sex.
- Use lubrication gel.
- Maintain a regular bowel care program.
- Avoid positions which caused autonomic hyperreflexia in the past.
- Ask your health care provider about medications to control the condition. If you already take medication, your health care provider may need to adjust your dosage.

Involuntary bowel movements

Sexual activity may cause an involuntary or unplanned bowel movement (incontinence). To avoid this, maintain a regular bowel care program or try to have a bowel movement before any sexual activity. To reduce the inconvenience of an unplanned bowel move-ment, place a collection container nearby and use a plastic mattress cover.

If you have had a colostomy or an ileostomy (surgical procedure done for bowel management), position your ostomy bag (used to collect stool after a colostomy or an ileostomy) out of the way. To prevent leakage during sexual activity:

- Use extra tape.
- Avoid direct pressure on the bag.
- Empty the bag before sexual activity.

For more information, see *Bowel Management*, Chapter Two.

Bladder leaks and catheter management

Sexual activity may cause urine to leak from your bladder. To avoid this, use your regular technique to empty your bladder before sexual activity. If you use a catheter, the following suggestions may assist in managing your catheter during sexual activity.

Indwelling catheter

For some people, it is unsafe to remove an indwelling catheter. If the catheter stays in place, wash your genitals before and after sexual activity. However, if your health care provider recommends removing the catheter:

- Be sure your bladder is empty before removing the catheter.
- Wash your genitals before and after sexual activity.
- After sexual activity, put in a sterile catheter.
- Do not leave the catheter out for longer than your health care provider recommends.

Considerations for males include:

- When you have an erection, bend the catheter over and along the shaft of your penis. Put a regular condom over it (Figure 8). A condom helps prevent the catheter from being dislodged from your bladder. Your penis and the catheter will fit into a woman's vagina.

Considerations for males and females include:

- Tape the drainage tube onto your abdomen (Figure 8).
- Place the drainage bag and tube out of the way.
- If your health care provider agrees, clamp the catheter and remove the bag for a short time.
- Use a water-soluble lubricant such as K-Y jelly™ to increase comfort.
- If you are concerned about leaks, keep towels close by.
- After sex, re-tape the catheter in the appropriate position for drainage.

Intermittent catheter

If you use an intermittent catheter:

- You may want to catheterize before sexual activity to make sure your bladder is empty.

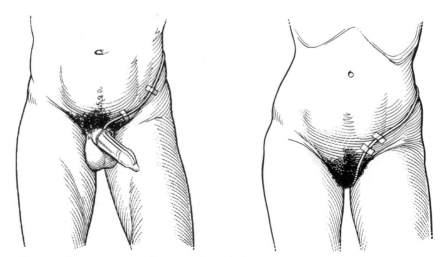

Figure 8. Drainage tube taped to abdomen.

- Wash your genitals before and after sexual activity.
- If you are concerned about leaks, keep towels close by.

External condom catheter

Considerations for an external condom catheter include:
- Before having intercourse, empty your bladder.
- Remove the condom catheter before sexual activity.
- Wash your genitals before and after sexual activity.
- In case of leaks, keep towels and a urinal close by.

Suprapubic catheter

If you use a suprabubic catheter:
- Be sure the catheter and drainage bag are out of the way.
- Wash your genitals before and after sexual activity.
- If you are concerned about leaks, keep towels close by.

Despite preparations, leaks may happen. You may want to keep towels at your bedside and consider a waterproof pad for your mattress. For more information, see Chapter Two, *Bladder Management*.

Medications

Medications taken for bladder problems and spasticity are those most likely to affect your sexual function. However, other medications can have an effect. These include medications prescribed for:
- Sleep
- Depression and anxiety
- Autonomic hyperreflexia (dysreflexia)
- High blood pressure

Some medications also affect your sexual response. If you are having a problem related to sexual response that you do not understand, talk to your health care provider. Continue to take your medications as directed. Discuss with your health care provider any concerns about how medications may affect your sexual function.

Endnote

Your spinal cord injury may affect your body's response to sexual stimuli. However, you are a sexual being with sexual desires. A fulfilling emotional and physical relationship is possible, but requires communication, experimentation and patience.

A professional counselor can be helpful to you in dealing with sexual issues. Your medical social worker and rehabilitation psychologist are trained in communication skills and counseling. Your health care provider can provide the medical information you need regarding sexual health. You can have a very satisfying future complete with intimacy and sexual pleasure.

Overcoming Limitations After a Spinal Cord Injury

6 Managing Your Independence

ESTABLISHING A RELATIONSHIP WITH A PERSONAL CARE ASSISTANT

You are establishing a relationship with a personal care assistant (PCA), who was hired to assist you with activities of daily living. Because this person works closely with you, it is important that both of you establish and maintain a good working relationship. This section provides information and tools that may be helpful in locating, interviewing and selecting a personal care assistant.

Employment Models

Before you proceed, you should know about the two different models for employing a personal care assistant — the agency model and the private pay model. In the agency model, a health care company (agency) employs the personal care assistant. In the private pay model, you, the consumer, are the employer.

Agency model

Assistance with your daily cares at home can be provided through various home care agencies. Some insurance companies may require the use of a Medicare certified agency for assistance. These agencies have a nurse that assures your care needs are identified and met.

Some agencies provide personal care assistance services only. Generally, if agencies are not Medicare certified (which is not a requirement for PCA services), they are required by the state to have qualified professionals assure that your care needs are met. Qualified professionals include registered nurses, psychologists (mental health provider), or licensed medical social workers.

The agency model can be used through some private insurance companies or if you qualify for Medicaid. The personal care assistant is an employee of the agency. You, as the consumer, must enroll with the agency providing the care and follow their guidelines. Even though the personal care assistant is employed by the agency, you might be involved in recruiting and interviewing applicants for the position.

Private pay model

In the private pay model, you are the employer. You pay the personal care assistant's salary. In addition to recruiting and interviewing, you hire, set the schedule and assign tasks for your personal care assistant. If you use this type of care model, you are responsible in assuring your needs are being met.

If you are not sure which model to use, talk with your social worker or a member of your health care team.

Needs Assessment

Regardless of the employment model, you should define your needs clearly before beginning the search for a personal care assistant. List all the activities that you may need help with. A checklist of possible activities is provided below. Go through this list and mark whether each activity is very important, somewhat important or not needed. If you need assistance with something that is not listed, write it down in a blank space.

Worksheet 1: Needs Assessment

Activity	Very Important	Somewhat Important	Not Needed
Bathing	❑	❑	❑
Grooming	❑	❑	❑
Dressing	❑	❑	❑
Skin/wound care	❑	❑	❑
Housekeeping			
• Daily	❑	❑	❑
• Weekly	❑	❑	❑
• Monthly	❑	❑	❑

Medications	❏	❏	❏
Range of motion/exercise	❏	❏	❏
Eating			
• Shopping	❏	❏	❏
• Preparing meals	❏	❏	❏
• Feeding	❏	❏	❏
• Cleanup	❏	❏	❏
Toilet			
• Bowel program	❏	❏	❏
• Bladder program	❏	❏	❏
• Other			
Transfers			
• Bed to wheelchair	❏	❏	❏
• Wheelchair to toilet	❏	❏	❏
• Shower	❏	❏	❏
• Tub	❏	❏	❏
• Other			
Wheelchair maintenance	❏	❏	❏
Recreation	❏	❏	❏
Errands	❏	❏	❏
Other	❏	❏	❏

As you identify activities requiring help, think about details such as how often and what time of day the activity needs to be done. Answers to these questions can help you decide if you need to hire more than one personal care assistant.

Next, you need to create a job description for the personal care assistant. This description should outline the specific requirements of the job and identify what skills and abilities your personal care assistant should have. The job description may also be called a task schedule or checklist for personal care.

This job description should be brief, step-by-step instructions for your personal care. It should include what needs to be done and the timing and sequence of steps. A well-written task schedule can be used as:
- A resource for questions when interviewing job applicants.
- Statement of your expectations of the personal care assistant.
- Definition of your role as the manager of your care.
- Flexible definition of your care needs.

Sample task schedule for morning routine
- [ ] 1. Get clothes ready
- [ ] 2. Prepare bathwater and materials needed for bathing
- [ ] 3. Check bathwater temperature
- [ ] 4. Assist in clothing removal
- [ ] 5. Move you from bed to bath
- [ ] 6. Wash and rinse body
- [ ] 7. Wash and rinse hair
- [ ] 8. Move you from bath to dressing area
- [ ] 9. Dry body thoroughly
- [ ] 10. Assist with dressing

As you create the job description, consider what you identified as needs on your needs assessment. In addition, think about:
- Skin care
- Equipment cleaning
- Respiratory assistance
- Turning and positioning
- Splints/braces/equipment
- Household cleaning tasks and routines

When listing qualifications and characteristics your personal care assistant should have, consider:
- Importance of previous similar experience
- Need for specialized training for your situation
- Need for driver's license/transportation
- Age, gender, etc., you will be most comfortable with
- Personality style preference, such as quiet and reserved or talkative and outgoing
- Time of day assistance is needed
- Essential skills, such as cooking, lifting, etc.
- Previous housekeeping experience
- Preference for someone who independently initiates work versus someone who needs direction from you
- Smoker versus non-smoker
- Promptness
- Reporting of absences
- Planning time off or vacations
- Other factors important to you

Think about areas that you consider important. Decide what areas are critical and where you can be flexible. Understanding the qualifications and characteristics that are most important to you, is vital to your choice of a personal care assistant.

Hiring Process

The first step in hiring a personal care assistant is advertising to recruit applicants. Different advertising approaches include:

- Advertising in a local newspaper or newsletter
- Checking with a health care company that might have a listing of available people
- Placing notices on bulletin boards
- Spreading the word through friends, family, churches or other organizations
- Checking Internet sites

Each approach can reach applicants. If your advertising is written or printed, make sure that the design of the ad or notice is attractive to the prospective employee. Place the information where it will be visible.

If you are advertising verbally, use all the opportunities available — family, friends, neighbors, classmates, co-workers, or other people you see informally.

Whatever your approach, provide enough information to attract qualified applicants. Your message should include:

- A brief description of the job
- Any special requirements
- The hours/days needed
- Salary
- Telephone number where applicants can reach you

The screening process begins as soon as an interested applicant contacts you. As you and the applicant introduce yourselves and begin to get acquainted, you should learn whether he or she meets the qualifications and can be considered for the job. At this point, you should describe the job, answer any questions and decide if the person is someone you might want to help you.

Based on your initial conversation, you can decide whether to proceed with a face-to-face interview. Before this interview, prepare questions that address the applicant's education, work experience, hobbies or interests, career plans and why the person is interested in this job. You will also want to discuss the work schedule, salary and a start date to see if they align with what you are expecting.

Sample interview questions
- "Why are you interested in this job?"
- "What past experiences have prepared you for this role?"

- "Tell me about a time when you and another person reached agreement, even though you may have had different opinions about something."
- "What kind of work schedule are you seeking?"
- "Describe a situation in which you had to acquire new skills and what you did to develop those skills."

If you are not working through an agency, you will need to check the applicant's references. However, if you are using an agency, they will do this for you. Checking references can help assure that the person has been truthful and reliable in reporting past experiences.

Even if you are pleased with the interview, it is generally not a good idea to hire someone "on the spot," especially if you are interviewing many candidates. Take time to think about the person's application, his or her responses to interview questions and your level of comfort with the applicant during the interview. Ask yourself if you would like this person working for you.

Once you have decided who to hire, call the applicant immediately to offer the position. After an applicant has accepted the position, notify other applicants the position has been filled. The last step in the hiring process is to create a "service agreement." This agreement should be tailored to your situation and may address the following areas:
- Duties
- Hours and work schedule
- Salary
- Use of personal items
- Policy on utilities
- Guidelines for smoking or alcohol use
- Behaviors that you consider unacceptable
- Responsibility for costs such as restaurant, taxi, etc.
- Termination notice

You will need to develop a backup plan in case you unexpectedly lose your personal care assistant's services. Consider family, agency and community resources that might be used to meet a short-term need.

Training Process

Training your personal care assistant is an ongoing process. If you are using an agency, the agency will provide your personal care assistant with general training. The agency's training will cover theoretical and practical information in several areas. However, since you may have unique needs and preferences, you should provide additional training to meet these needs. The agency will also provide the personal care assistant with information about communication techniques and employee policies. If you are not using an agency, this training will be your responsibility.

You may want to have the new personal care assistant spend some time with you while another person who is used to helping you is present. By doing so, your new personal care assistant gets hands-on experience and a chance to learn by seeing and doing. Make sure your new personal care assistant goes through daily routines and procedures. You may want the person to demonstrate procedures after observing them being done.

On the worksheet below, identify the areas in which your personal care assistant needs information unique to your situation.

Worksheet 2: Training Needs
- ❏ Types of disabilities or disabling conditions
- ❏ Nutrition
- ❏ Infection control
- ❏ Skin care
- ❏ Bowel management
- ❏ Bladder management
- ❏ Transfer techniques (to and from a wheelchair, bed, etc.)
- ❏ Range of motion/exercise management
- ❏ Management of the home
- ❏ Activities of daily living
- ❏ Other

During this time of on-the-job learning, create a relaxed and open environment. Let your new personal care assistant know that you will answer questions. The assistant may be curious about your physical condition, equipment you use, or the arrangement of your home environment.

You should clearly explain to your new personal care assistant about what you can and cannot do and how much help you expect. This openness lays the groundwork for creating a true "team spirit" between you and your personal care assistant. This "team spirit" contributes to the healthy working relationship that is essential for overcoming any challenges in the future.

MANAGING AND DIRECTING YOUR DAILY CARE

You (the consumer), your personal care assistant and the qualified professional, together will manage your daily activities. It is important to be comfortable with the qualified professional and personal care assistant involved in your care. The qualified professional should work with you to see that your care needs are identified and met through the use of available resources.

This section discusses the role of the qualified professional and personal care assistant, as well as guidelines and skills for managing your personal care assistant and other aspects of your care.

The Consumer, Qualified Professional and Personal Care Assistant Roles

Your role as the consumer includes:
- Working with the qualified professional to define your personal care needs and a plan.
- Completion of a job description for your personal care assistant.
- Recruitment and selection of your personal care assistant.
- Setting a realistic work schedule for your personal care assistant.
- Notifying the qualified professional if your name, address or telephone number changes.
- Reporting changes in your condition or care needs.

The role of the qualified professional includes:
- Assessing your personal care needs.
- Developing a plan of care with you.
- Hiring and training your personal care assistant.
- Supervising the care given by the personal care assistant.
- Processing forms for governmental payment programs (such as Medicaid).

The role of the personal care assistant includes:
- Providing care as outlined in the job description.
- Reporting changes in your condition (such as a skin breakdown) to the qualified professional.
- Completing and filing reports with the agency (if you are using one) detailing the time worked and care provided.

Managing Your Personal Care Assistant

You and your personal care assistant must have a healthy working relationship. Both of you must understand your roles and responsibilities in order to manage your care effectively. Because you and your personal care assistant work closely together, roles can easily become confused unless you use effective methods to manage and maintain good relationships.

State your expectations and delegate tasks clearly to your personal care assistant—be specific and direct. Then, confirm that your personal care assistant understands. If something is not done as you requested, think about whether the difference is important. If it is important, talk again with the personal care assistant about your preferences. Be open-minded about new or different approaches to doing things. Remember that you are both human and make mistakes.

Above all, clear, concise and frequent communication of employment expectations for your personal care assistant is critical to the success of the relationship. You cannot communicate too much. Share information, ask and answer questions, provide feedback and talk with each other.

The following helpful reminders may ensure effective communication between you and your personal care assistant:

- *Make no assumptions:* Communicate specific details verbally or in writing until the task is completed or you are sure that your personal care assistant understands.
- *Answer questions:* Clear and concise responses given patiently assure that you and your personal care assistant know your care needs and how to meet them.
- *Use checklists and other written reminders:* Written information clarifies your expectations and assures that the same steps or actions will be done each time.
- *Explain why tasks are done a certain way:* Explanations may provide your personal care assistant with a better understanding of your preferences.
- *Expect mistakes:* Nobody's perfect.
- *Offer praise as well as constructive feedback:* Effective feedback reinforces the positive aspects of your personal care assistant's work and allows for changes in care where needed.
- *Treat your personal care assistant as you would like to be treated:* With respect and courtesy. You both may have days when you feel upbeat as well as days when you feel "blue."

Other Aspects of Your Daily Care Management

Finances

If your personal care assistant is employed by an agency (the agency model), the agency pays your assistant. If you are using the private pay model, you are the employer. You are responsible for recruiting, hiring, firing, paying wages and reporting the payment of cash and non cash wages for tax purposes. In this situation, you may want to consult a tax adviser for information about tax laws and your obligations as an employer.

Ongoing education

Initially, general training for your personal care assistant will be handled by the agency involved and you will provide training specific to your personal needs. Beyond this initial training, you may need to provide ongoing training.

As your needs and preferences change, you will want to make sure that your personal care assistant has the appropriate information and skills to meet your needs. Communicate clearly with your personal care assistant and with the qualified professional if additional training is needed.

Record keeping

If you are using the agency model, you will have minimal responsibilities for record keeping. Your personal care assistant will complete a time sheet noting time spent with you. You must sign this time sheet after verifying it is correct. This allows you to accurately keep track of the hours used as part of the total number of allowed hours.

If you are using the private pay model, you will have the record keeping responsibilities associated with being an employer. In this case, you may want to consult a business adviser for information about record keeping for employment and tax purposes.

Confidentiality

Your personal care assistant needs to know what information about you should be confidential. Since the workplace is also your home environment, you must both respect the other's personal property and right to privacy. Agree in advance what your personal care assistant's role will be in discussions of personal issues. Use the following answers to questions to help you reach an agreement:

- Do you expect your personal care assistant to listen, to share opinions, to identify resources or to suggest alternatives?
- How do your expectations compare to what your personal care assistant feels comfortable doing?

Confidentiality must be addressed early in the working relationship to decrease the chance of any misunderstandings later.

Directing Your Care

Directing your personal care assistant how to meet your care needs requires skill. The most important skills you will need are active listening, assertiveness, and giving and receiving feedback.

Active listening

Active listening is a skill that must be learned and practiced. It is easy to hear the words but not the message. You may be preoccupied with your own message or distracted by your thoughts or feelings and not listen closely enough to understand. The following guidelines may help you practice good active listening skills with those involved in your care.

- Focus on the person who is talking. Show interest in the speaker's message by establishing and maintaining eye contact as you listen. An occasional nod, your facial expression, body position or gestures can show that you are truly interested and attentive to the message.
- Try to understand the speaker's viewpoint by considering the values, beliefs and assumptions that might affect the message. Ask yourself if the message is about facts or feelings. When in doubt, ask a question or restate what you thought you heard to clarify or confirm the speaker's actual message.
- Think about your values, beliefs and assumptions that may influence your ability to listen. Avoid jumping to conclusions or thinking about your response while the other person is still talking. Don't plan your response or make up your mind until you are certain that you have heard and understood the entire message.
- Work at being a good listener. Hearing requires no effort from you. But really listening to a message means making an effort to pay close attention and understand what you hear.

Assertiveness

Assertiveness is another essential communication skill necessary in directing your care.

Assertive communication

Assertive communication allows you to share the thoughts and opinions that reflect your best interests without hurting the other person's feelings. Assertiveness is standing up for your own rights while not imposing on the rights of others.

Passive communication

Passive or nonassertive communication means not expressing your feelings and ideas and giving in to others. As a result, you often feel misunderstood or believe that others take advantage of you.

Aggressive communication

Aggressive communication means sharing your feelings and ideas in a way that hurts and offends others. As a result, you may get your point across, but you may be seen as a critical, thoughtless person.

Assertive communication is more effective than either passive or aggressive communication. If you are assertive, you speak about a need or problem honestly and directly and still feel good about yourself. The person who is listening receives the message and still feels respected as a person. This promotes an effective working relationship as you both participate as equals in dealing with the need or problem.

Feedback

Feedback means communicating to another person about his or her actions in order to help evaluate behavior. Feedback is an important skill to have when working with a personal care assistant. You can use feedback to clarify ideas and expectations, increase understanding and find ways to change things that need to be changed.

Feedback should be positive or constructive. Both types are essential in a healthy working relationship. If you only provide positive feedback, you both miss chances to improve your skills. If you only provide constructive feedback, your personal care assistant may become discouraged.

Positive feedback

Positive feedback recognizes a person's strengths or contributions. Both the giver and the receiver of the feedback feel good. Positive feedback can tell the personal care assistant what tasks or activities are being done well. Your personal care assistant also realizes that you appreciate the efforts made in your care.

Here are some tips for giving positive feedback:

- *Be spontaneous and sincere:* Share your comments as soon as you notice something done well.
- *Be specific:* "You always gather all the things I'll need for my shower and set the water temperature just as I like it." That statement is more effective than the general comment, "You do a great job with my shower."
- Realize that others appreciate your opinion and benefit from your praise.
- *Put it in writing:* The feedback will last longer.
- *Make it a habit:* Consistently acknowledge work that is done well.

Constructive feedback

Constructive feedback provides a person with information that can be used to change behavior. You can share constructive feedback to inform your personal care assistant about tasks or activities that are not done as you expect. This feedback benefits both of you. It allows you to express concerns about your care honestly but objectively. The personal care assistant becomes aware of your opinion and has the opportunity to change the behavior. As with positive feedback, constructive feedback must be specific and timely.

Here are some tips for giving constructive feedback:

- Focus on the behavior and how that behavior affects you.
- Constructive feedback should never be used to release anger or hostility, or to make the other person feel guilty, stupid or worthless.

The REAP method

The REAP method is one approach to giving feedback. This method may help you give constructive feedback to a personal care assistant.

- **REPORT** what happened without judgment. Share the fact, not your ideas about why something happened, or what the meaning or intent was. Focus on the specific action, not the person.
- **EXPRESS** the impact the action had on you. Focus on how you were affected or how you felt as a result of what the person did or did not do. Calmly share your thoughts and feelings using "I" statements.
- **ASK** for what you want. Clarify what you expect. Think about what changes you would consider an improvement and then explore ways to make those changes happen. Be sure that what you ask for is reasonable.

- State the **PAYOFFS** for both of you. Describe both the rewards for change and the consequences of not changing. Decide what is negotiable in the payoff.

Effectively communicating with your personal care assistant is important but can be surprisingly complex. The three skills of active listening, assertiveness and feedback will help you communicate with your personal care assistant in a way that benefits both of you. Practice these skills, because if you use them often, you should become more skilled at them. The result will be a healthy working relationship that will have positive outcomes for everyone involved.

MAINTAINING AN EFFECTIVE RELATIONSHIP WITH A PERSONAL CARE ASSISTANT

Your relationship with your personal care assistant is important. You may spend more time with your personal care assistant than with any other member of the health care team. At times, the effectiveness of this relationship may be threatened by conflict. Even in the best working relationships, conflicts may arise.

Since human relationships are complex, it is not surprising that the potential for problems and conflict exists. When conflict occurs, it is important that both you and your personal care assistant face the problem directly and promptly. If you are not comfortable dealing with the issue on your own, find an advocate to work with you and your personal care assistant to solve the problem. Don't let issues pile up, or both you and your personal care assistant may become frustrated and angry, and end the relationship without giving it a proper chance to succeed.

What is Conflict?

Conflict can be defined as a disagreement. It occurs when one person's wants or needs do not agree with someone else's. In your case, the other person in the conflict would be your personal care assistant.

Conflict can result from wrong assumptions, different expectations, unclear communication, questions about personal boundaries, or conflicting beliefs or values. For example, if your personal care assistant does not perform a task to your satisfaction, you can ask several questions to determine why:

- Has one of you made a wrong assumption?
- Does the personal care assistant's job description clearly list the expectations for this task?
- Have you explained clearly how and why to complete the task?
- Have you and your personal care assistant discussed each of your roles in completing this task?
- Do you and your personal care assistant disagree about the importance or value of the task?

Answering these questions may help you discover why the conflict occurred. Determining why may help you and your personal care assistant deal with the conflict.

Strategies for Success

One of the most effective ways to maintain a good working relationship with your personal care assistant is to communicate clearly. Active listening, assertiveness and feedback are key skills in sending and receiving messages clearly. At times, however, even if you think you have used these skills, a misunderstanding may occur. When this happens, review your written and oral messages first, to see if anything is missing.

If unclear or missing communication does not seem to be the source of your problem, consider addressing the problem by:
- Boundary setting
- Problem solving
- Conflict resolution

Each strategy can help you maintain a good relationship with your personal care assistant.

Boundary setting

Boundary setting means clearly defining the limits in the working relationship between you and your personal care assistant. The service agreement that was completed when your personal care assistant was hired should have included general information about what is expected of him or her. Specific information about each of your responsibilities in meeting your care needs should have been outlined in the job description or task schedule.

For example, if you expect your personal care assistant to be available if you ask for help with a specific task, but not to do the task for you, both of you should clearly understand your responsibilities. If a problem arises because boundaries have not been clearly defined or understood, you and your personal care assistant may need to discuss and clarify the task schedule or service agreement.

Problem solving

Problem solving can be used to make decisions that will correct, improve, or enhance a situation to satisfy the people involved. Try problem solving if you are concerned about your care or the behavior of your personal care assistant in providing that care.

Listed below are some helpful hints to remember when problem solving:
- Focus on the problem not the person.
- Look for many possible solutions rather than a single answer.
- Remember that your goal is to find the best solution rather than to be right.
- Find ways to cooperate, not compete, with your personal care assistant.

The problem solving process consists of five steps. They are listed below, along with a brief description of what you and your personal care assistant should do.

Step 1: State the problem
Explain the problem to your personal care assistant. Use your communication skills to make sure that he or she understands that you think a problem exists. Look at all aspects of the problem and share your concerns with one another.

Step 2: Define the problem
Be specific about your concerns. Consider your side of the situation and also your personal care assistant's viewpoint. You and your personal care assistant should discuss the situation thoroughly to determine the real issue. It is necessary that you agree a problem exists, define the problem, and set a goal for solving the problem.

Step 3: Consider possible solutions
Think of all the possible actions that may be used to solve the problem. Your goal is to come up with as many ideas as possible. You and your personal care assistant may both make suggestions as you discuss ideas. Since you want to have as many solutions as possible, do not eliminate any ideas at this point. Keep track of them until you get to the next step of the process.

Step 4: Evaluate possible choices
Once you have identified different approaches to solving the problem, you can decide which approach is best. Think about your beliefs and values, which reflect what is most important to you and help provide direction.

Next, you and your personal care assistant should consider the strengths and weaknesses related to each solution. Doing this can help you decide which approach would be easier and which would be more difficult. After this step, you should have a clearer idea of the best solution.

Step 5: Choose a solution
You are ready to select the best solution in light of your values, beliefs, strengths and weaknesses. If you and your personal care assistant have communicated clearly and honestly throughout the problem solving process, you should be ready to make a choice. You will know that you have:
- Identified the right problem.
- Shared your views of the problem.
- Listed possible ways to solve the problem.
- Discussed each possibility to decide if the solution might work.
- Considered your most important values and beliefs.
- Recognized the strengths and weaknesses of each possible solution.
- Chosen the best way to try to solve the problem.

Try the solution you chose and see if you have corrected, improved or enhanced the situation to satisfy both you and your personal care assistant. If you think you can do even better, repeat the process with any new information you have.

Conflict resolution

If problem solving does not correct, improve or enhance a situation to satisfy those involved, you may need to try conflict resolution. Conflict resolution is a way to address an ongoing problem that threatens to end the working relationship.

The main goal of conflict resolution is to successfully resolve the problem. In addition, you and your personal care assistant should end up feeling like winners. The following tips may help you to achieve both goals when resolving a conflict.

Determine the "real" source of conflict

Four types of conflict exist:
- *Information conflict:* Happens when the people involved act a certain way because they do not have the same information.
- *Values conflict:* Occurs when people have different priorities or beliefs because their values are different.
- *Personality conflict:* Is rare, but happens when personality traits are so different that the people involved just can't seem to get along.
- *Style conflict:* Is created when the people involved have different ways of approaching tasks, work or life in general.

Deciding which type of conflict is present can lead to choosing the best way to resolve it. The key is determining the "real" source of conflict.

To find the "real" source, think about the answers to these questions:
- When did the conflict start?
- Who is involved besides you and your personal care assistant (if anyone)?
- What information do you have?
- What information do you need?
- What information does your personal care assistant have?
- What information does your personal care assistant need?
- What emotions are involved?
- Are feelings of rivalry, competition, power or control present?

The answers to these questions can help you identify the "real" source of the conflict. Then, you can decide how to proceed.

"C" the way to manage the conflict

You might use one of four different approaches to resolve the conflict:
- Compromise
- Collaboration
- Confrontation
- Creative avoidance

Compromise
Compromise means that the people involved in the conflict try to find common ground to reach a joint decision. Compromise is based on cooperation. However, some people may feel that compromise may require them to set aside their own beliefs or give up something. In this situation, compromise may be seen as a win-lose or lose-win situation.

Collaboration

Collaboration involves working together so that all points of view and information are shared and heard. Those in conflict consider the concerns of all and look for a solution that pleases everyone. This approach reflects a win-win situation and is the best approach to maintain or improve the working relationship.

Confrontation

Confrontation points out inconsistencies between a person's words and actions. This approach may be used if power, control or other issues are causing the conflict. In confrontation, people communicate the differences between what people say and what they do. The person being confronted has a chance to change his or her behavior to improve the working relationship.

Creative avoidance

In creative avoidance, the people involved find ways to avoid dealing with the conflict and still share the same world. Since you and your personal care assistant must spend a lot of time together, and you rely on him or her to help with your care, this is probably not a very effective approach to consider.

If conflict is not resolved

There are times when, despite your best efforts, the problems in your relationship become more than you can handle by yourself. You may have tried to resolve conflict using the methods described in this material, but still, you need to make a change.

If this happens, talk with a member of your health care team about how to begin the process of terminating your personal care assistant. People who can help include a registered nurse, a mental health provider, or a licensed social worker. These qualified professionals can give you advice about how to terminate the personal care assistant.

Terminating the personal care assistant

Informing the assistant

As your assistant's employer, it is your responsibility to inform the assistant that he or she is terminated. You can tell the assistant in person or in writing. If you terminate the assistant in person, have a trustworthy person with you as a witness. Use open, honest communication about when and why. If you do so in writing, be sure to keep a copy.

Final payment

Make arrangement before terminating your assistant how you will pay any wages you owe him or her. Keep detailed records as proof of final payment.

When to terminate

How quickly you terminate the personal care assistant depends on how serious the problems are in your relationship. If you feel the reasons are not serious, that is, they are not harmful to you; it may be a good idea to give your assistant notice. Less serious reasons include you just aren't getting along, or you don't like the way the assistant performs a certain caregiving task. Typically, employers give employees notice ranging from a couple days to a couple weeks.

If you give notice, use the time to look for a new assistant. You may not find an assistant who is going to be a long-term solution, but one that can fill in until then. Be sure to consider the differences in cost of care when changing to a different assistant. Plan ahead so you can budget for the differences in cost.

Sometimes, the reason you need to terminate the employee is very serious. For example, the assistant may be hurting or neglecting you. If this is the case, follow these guidelines:

- Report what has happened to your local police department or call 9-1-1. Tell the assistant you have done so.
- When you inform the assistant that his or her employment is being terminated, consider your personal safety. Either do so over the phone, or, if in person, have someone with you.

The basic process for terminating your assistant should be detailed in the service agreement explained earlier in this material. If you need help completing any forms related to termination, have other questions about the process, or concerns about your safety, ask a qualified professional for help.

Abuse, Neglect, Fraud, and Exploitation

If you feel you are the victim of abuse or fraud, contact your local police department, call 9-1-1, or your county's human services department. To help determine if this is the case, it may help to understand what these terms really mean.

Abuse is when a person is purposefully injured, either physically, mentally or emotionally. Abuse can be an act of direct harm or an act of omission that leads to harm. Examples can include grabbing you, yelling at you, or encouraging someone else to harm you.

Neglect is failure to provide adequate food, shelter, affection, supervision or medical care on a regular basis. Examples include your assistant regularly not giving you enough food or ignoring your health care needs.

Fraud is when someone tricks you, deceives you, or cheats you. It is done intentionally and is used to get you to give up something that is legally yours such as money or your rights. An example might be that an assistant convinces you that you are not capable of handing your own money, and gets you to sign over your bank account, then takes money from your account.

Exploitation is when someone takes advantage of you in some way in order to make things better for him or herself. An example might be your assistant regularly borrows your personal belongings such as your clothes or your car.

As a person with a spinal cord injury, you may be in a vulnerable position. Some people may think it is easy to take advantage of you. Be aware of people asking personal questions such as ones about your financial situation or family details. Talk to someone you trust such as a family member or good friend if you are not sure of something.

Remember, if you feel your personal care assistant has neglected you, taken advantage of you, or that you have been the victim of fraud or exploitation, call 9-1-1, or tell a member of your health care team. Others can help and you do not have to manage alone.

UNDERSTANDING THE NEEDS OF THE FAMILY CAREGIVER

You have decided to involve a family member (such as a spouse, parent, or adult child) or a friend in your care. This person may work as an employee and receive pay, or may help on an unpaid basis. This involvement in your care can be helpful since you already know each other and have a good idea of how to get along. Understanding your caregiver's needs is important.

Needs of the Family Caregiver

The caregiver role

If the person assisting with your care is a paid personal care assistant, use the same process you would if they were not a family member or friend. However, if the person providing your care is not being paid as a personal care assistant, they may be referred to as a caregiver. Even though your caregiver is not being paid, most of the principles used in a working relationship with a personal care assistant still apply.

You both must know what your care needs are and what is expected of the caregiver to meet those needs. You must also decide what training is needed to meet your care needs. You will want to discuss confidentiality and any other areas that might create problems when you work with a family member or friend. Create forms such as a task schedule, job description, or service agreement. These forms will explain clearly what you both expect in your working relationship.

Your caregiver may also have other roles, such as being a spouse, parent or child in the family, and may have a job or other responsibilities outside the home. Therefore, your caregiver may feel as if he or she is constantly "on duty" or expected to do it all. Your caregiver will need to balance their time and energy to fulfill all these roles.

Needs of the caregiver

Generally, caregivers have four types of needs:
- Physical
- Emotional
- Spiritual
- Financial

Physical needs
Physical needs include rest and sleep, physical and mental exercise, a well-balanced diet, and other behaviors to maintain good health.

Adequate rest on a regular basis is important so that your caregiver has the energy and alertness to provide your care. If a full night's sleep is not possible, work with your caregiver to set up a plan for naps or break periods during the day.

Your caregiver should take time for physical exercise and conditioning activities. Doing these activities on a regular basis may increase his or her strength, reduce injury, allow for better rest, and enhance his or her ability to provide your care. Talk with your caregiver about a plan for physical exercise and conditioning. Think about setting aside a certain time during the day when your caregiver can exercise, or suggest the use of certain times during the daily routine as a chance for physical activity.

Mental exercise is just as important as physical exercise. It helps your caregiver to be alert. Allow time in your daily routine to find out about current events and news. Spending time reading newspapers or magazines, scanning informative Internet sites or watching television news programs can provide helpful information to broaden both of your views.

Other mental exercises such as reading, puzzles, and board and card games, may help to provide your caregiver with mental exercise. These activities may be a welcome change of pace and a source of pleasure. Even social conversations with friends, family members or neighbors can be refreshing and thought provoking.

Your caregiver should eat a well-balanced diet. At times, your caregiver may not feel like eating or may not think that there is time to eat a proper diet. However, healthy, nutritious meals are an important part of assuring that your caregiver has enough energy.

Finally, your caregiver must take care of his or her general health. Regular visits to a health care provider can prevent problems or detect them early. Your caregiver should immediately report any illness or other health problems to a health care provider, so they can be treated right away. If your caregiver is sick, both of you are affected.

Emotional needs
Emotional needs include support, reassurance, ways to cope, and leisure activities. These needs must be met since they are closely associated with physical health.

Like everyone, caregivers need support and reassurance. They may experience many confusing or conflicting feelings. For example, they may feel joyful and sorrowful, hopeful and hopeless, happy and sad. Though your caregiver may try to label these feelings as "good" or "bad", feelings such as these are normal.

Caregivers should admit their feelings and find a support system to deal with them. Having a close friend or family member whom they can call often may help. You might encourage your caregiver to consider joining an organization or support group for caregivers. Other possible sources of support and reassurance may include social workers, clergy, or counselors. Your caregiver should learn how to ask for help when needed.

Your caregiver also needs to find ways to deal with the frustration, tension or irritation that they feel at times. If your caregiver already has a method that works, he or she should continue to use it. If not, you and your caregiver might discuss this need. Ask your caregiver to consider using various techniques for coping such as taking a walk, housecleaning, talking to friends or family or other similar activities. A sense of humor may also help to deal with feelings.

Finding a regular way to cope with feelings can help meet your caregiver's emotional needs.

Spiritual needs

Spiritual needs include inner peace and strength. Many activities that help meet physical and emotional needs also support spiritual health. Your caregiver's spiritual needs may be met by a brief quiet time during the day. Relaxation exercises or visiting a relaxing place like a park or river, reading from prayer reflection books or listening to music are other ways for your caregiver to find some peace. Your caregiver should choose an approach they enjoy and use it to maintain their spiritual strength.

Financial needs

Financial needs include those related to the cost of providing care for someone. Income and expenses may change for the person providing care as well as for the rest of the family.

Discuss financial changes with your caregiver to help determine what is necessary to meet those needs. Potential costs to consider include:
- Lost income
- A change in pension or other benefits
- Impact of spending on a fixed income
- Changes at home, such as remodeling or relocating
- Medical costs
- Housekeeping or home maintenance expenses

These needs must be compared to available financial resources. Your caregiver may wish to talk with a financial advisor to plan ways to meet their financial needs.

So how can your caregiver meet his or her needs and still have the time to provide your care?

To make sure your caregiver has time to provide your care and still have their needs met, he or she may wish to combine activities to achieve a balance. For example, a daily walk with a friend may provide physical exercise and support. Time spent with a reading group may be thought-provoking, socially entertaining and peaceful.

If your caregiver feels too overwhelmed to address all these needs at once, they should decide to start by working on one or two of the most important needs. Your caregiver must set realistic goals and work toward those goals. You should support your caregiver in all efforts to stay physically, mentally, emotionally and financially healthy so that they are better able to provide your care.

Respite care

Even if you and your caregiver follow the advice above, your caregiver may still need to take a break from the responsibilities of providing your care. Therefore, your caregiver may need to plan time to get away, a respite, which may last a day or longer. This time can be spent in any manner your caregiver wishes, such as spending time alone or with friends. It can also be used for relaxing or for trying new activities.

Sometimes your caregiver may not wish to take a break, because they may:
- Want to be the only one involved in your care
- Feel that your care is a duty
- Believe that they have all the skills necessary to provide your care
- Feel that no one else understands your needs as well as they do
- Think that no one else would be able to provide the same quality of care
- Feel that you don't want anyone else involved in your care

Although some of these statements may be true, you should consider that it may be best to involve others in your care for short periods so that your family member or friend can continue providing your care long term.

If your caregiver plans to be away for an extended period of time, you may need to find someone who can fill in for your caregiver (respite care). Like other aspects of your care, arranging respite care involves careful planning. Think about the answers to the following questions:
- Do you want respite care regularly, for example, on the same evening each week or the same time each day?
- What activities will you expect the substitute caregiver to help with?

If you are planning respite care, you and your caregiver must decide what type of help you need. Be specific and consider each detail of your care in the following areas:
- Personal care
- Housekeeping
- Meal preparation
- Transportation
- Medical care
- Recreation

- Shopping
- Companionship

Involve other family members and friends. They may want a chance to help even if they have not offered in the past. Ask a clergy member, social worker, or health care provider for ideas about people who might help. Other possible ideas may come from local United Way agencies, hospitals, churches, or referral centers. Decide what financial resources you can use to provide this help, such as assistance from local agencies that offer services.

If you are unsure about having someone new involved in providing your care, discuss this with your caregiver. You and your caregiver can then plan to make sure you feel comfortable with respite care. For example, your respite caregiver could observe your caregiver providing your care. This would allow the three of you to spend time together.

The person helping you will need to know your routine and what is expected. They will also need to know how to reach your caregiver if a problem occurs. You and your caregiver should discuss any other details that you think the respite caregiver needs to know.

If you are using respite care for the first time, consider a "trial run" so all those involved can see how it works. If the care provided is not perfect the first time, don't give up. Think about what worked and changes to make when you use respite care again. Above all, remember that the purpose of respite care is to give your caregiver a break so they can return with renewed energy to help you.

7 Staying Healthy After Spinal Cord Injury

NUTRITION

What you eat (nutrition) contributes to your physical and mental health and helps your body fight infection and disease. Getting the right nutrients in adequate amounts can help you maintain good health.

The purpose of this chapter is to help you understand the importance of good nutrition following a spinal cord injury. This includes identifying factors that may contribute to poor nutrition, as well as understanding the best sources for nutrients and goals of nutritional management.

Poor Nutrition

Poor nutrition means you are not eating enough healthy food. Following SCI, certain factors can contribute to poor nutrition. These may include:
- Injury or trauma
- Trouble feeding yourself
- Trouble swallowing
- Irregular bowel and bladder habits
- Depression

If you lose your appetite, some changes may help. One way is to choose pleasant surroundings to eat in and invite someone to join you. You may also find it easier to eat smaller meals more often. If swallowing is a problem, eat soft, easy-to-chew foods. If you cannot eat enough, milkshakes or other high-calorie or protein drinks can help.

Poor nutrition may also occur with overeating, if you eat foods high in calories and low in nutritional value (candy, cookies, soda and chips). Avoid food with poor nutritional value. A dietitian can help you make healthy food choices. An occupational therapist can provide aids such as special utensils and cups if you need help eating.

Signs of poor nutrition

Early signs of poor nutrition may include:
- General weakness and fatigue
- Irritability
- Decreased attention span
- Dry skin
- Significant weight loss or weight gain
- Poor healing of wounds or incisions

Source and Purpose of Nutrients

Table 1 lists essential nutrients, the foods (source) that contain them and their purpose. A dietitian can help you determine the right serving and portion size needed for each nutrient.

Protein

Proteins, which are essential to human life, are contained in every cell in your body. Proteins build and repair body structures, carry nutrients to your cells and regulate body processes. After SCI, you may need more protein. Getting enough protein is essential to maintain good health, promote healing and prevent infection.

At each meal, choose a good source of protein. Aim for 1 to 2 ounces of protein at breakfast and 2 to 3 ounces of protein at lunch and at dinner. In general, one serving of protein equals:
- 3 ounces of meat, poultry or fish (about the size of a deck of cards)
- ½ cup cooked dry beans
- 1 egg
- 2 tablespoons of peanut butter
- ½ cup of nuts or seeds

If you have **pressure ulcers** or an infection, your protein needs will likely be even higher. Talk to a dietitian to help you determine how much protein you need.

Table 1 Nutrients

Nutrient	Source	Purpose
Major nutrients		
Protein	Milk and milk products, meat, poultry, fish, eggs and meat alternatives.	To build, repair and maintain muscle, nerves and other tissues.
Simple carbohydrates	Fruits, honey and milk.	To supply energy.
Complex carbohydrates	Whole grains, bran products, fresh fruits and vegetables.	To provide fiber and help regulate bowel function.
Fats	Meat and meat alternatives, whole milk and dairy products, margarines and oils.	Act as a source of energy, protect and insulate the body, promote normal growth and development.
Other nutrients		
Vitamins (e.g., A, B, C, D, E, K)	Found in a variety of foods. Talk to a dietitian for more information.	Play an important role in metabolism (the physical and chemical changes that make energy for your body to use), promote normal energy, growth and development, help prevent infection.
Minerals (e.g., calcium, phosphorus, iron, potassium, sodium)	Found in a variety of foods. Talk to a dietitian for more information.	Control many chemical mechanisms in the body, such as fluid balance and blood volume, make bones and teeth strong, affect regulation of muscular and nervous system.
Water	All beverages, fruits and vegetables.	To help digest and eliminate wastes from the body, regulate body temperature, make all body functions possible.

Carbohydrates

Carbohydrates can be simple or complex. Simple carbohydrates are the sugars found in fruits, honey and milk. The body absorbs them quickly for energy. Complex carbohydrates, also known as starches, are found primarily in whole grains, pasta, potatoes, beans and vegetables. They contain many vitamins and minerals as well as fiber and help regulate bowel function.

Fiber

There are two types of dietary fiber—soluble and insoluble.
- *Soluble fiber:* Increases stool volume and may play a role in lowering cholesterol. Food sources of soluble fiber include oats,

barley, and some fruits and vegetables (citrus fruits, peaches, plums, carrots, broccoli, beans and peas).
- *Insoluble fiber:* Stimulates the intestine and increases stool mass, preventing constipation. Wheat bran, whole-grain breads and cereals, brown rice, and some fruits and vegetables (apples, pears with the skin, broccoli and spinach) contain high levels of insoluble fiber.

Since different types of fiber have different functions in the body, choosing a variety of high-fiber foods is important.

Fats

Certain fats are essential to the life and function of the body's cells. Along with providing reserves of stored energy, these fats affect the immune system and help regulate many body processes. Deposits of fat tissues protect and insulate vital body organs. Therefore, some fat is essential in your diet. The healthiest fats are monosaturated fats, found in nuts, avocados, canola oil, olive oil and peanut oil.

Fluids

You will need to increase your fluid intake following SCI. Fluids are especially important during wound healing. Since all healing and maintenance of bodily functions require fluid, too little fluid results in slower healing.

Drink 8 to 10 cups of caffeine-free beverages every day. Drinking beverages with caffeine will cause you to lose as much fluid as you are consuming. Water is the best choice. Some foods such as popsi-cles®, ice cream and watermelon can count as beverages since their fluid content is high (½ cup serving equals approximately 4 ounces of fluid).

Watch the color of your urine to help determine if you are drinking enough fluid (pale yellow color is ideal). During the hot summer months your fluid needs are higher since you lose fluid by perspiring. If you are on a fluid schedule or fluid restriction, discuss your fluid needs with your health care provider.

Nutritional Management

The goals of nutritional management following SCI are:
- *To maximize nutritional intake:* Your body needs nutrients to provide energy. Nutrients also build, repair and maintain the body. To function well, your body needs protein, carbohydrates, fats,

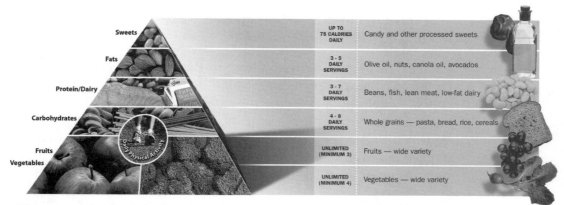

Sweets	UP TO 75 CALORIES DAILY	Candy and other processed sweets
Fats	3 - 5 DAILY SERVINGS	Olive oil, nuts, canola oil, avocados
Protein/Dairy	3 - 7 DAILY SERVINGS	Beans, fish, lean meat, low-fat dairy
Carbohydrates	4 - 8 DAILY SERVINGS	Whole grains — pasta, bread, rice, cereals
Fruits	UNLIMITED (MINIMUM 3)	Fruits — wide variety
Vegetables	UNLIMITED (MINIMUM 4)	Vegetables — wide variety

Figure 1. The food guide pyramid. A guide to daily food choices.

vitamins, minerals and water. A good diet should include food from all major food groups (Figure 1). The goal of a balanced diet is to ensure adequate calories to maintain a healthy weight, while getting the nutrients your body needs.

- *To maintain a healthy weight:* When an SCI first occurs, you may lose weight, perhaps because of your body's additional need for calories and nutrients during healing. However, about one year after your injury, weight gain can become a problem because you need fewer calories. Typically, the reason is due to a change in your activity level.

How your weight is distributed also changes. The amount of muscle decreases and the amount of fat tends to increase. What and how much you eat will need to be adjusted immediately after your injury and periodically thereafter. This adjustment can help you reach and maintain your desired weight. Persons with SCI who are overweight or underweight are at risk for complications such as skin breakdown, constipation and respiratory infections.

- *To help regulate your bladder and bowel habits:* People with SCI need to drink appropriate amounts of fluid to assist with bladder function. The amount of fluid you will need is generally based on your bladder management program. Diet is also important in regulating your bowel movements.

FITNESS

A person who is physically fit has a greater ability to resist illness and injury, and to recover faster from an illness. Physical fitness includes exercising your heart and lungs (cardiovascular system), and muscles. Physical wellness includes exercising your body and mind to benefit your overall health.

Exercise helps reduce the buildup of deposits in your arteries by increasing the concentration of high density lipoprotein (HDL or "good") cholesterol (a fatlike substance) in your blood, thus reducing your risk of cardiovascular disease. Exercise also strengthens your heart so that it can pump blood more efficiently and supply oxygen and nutrients throughout the body. Your heart, lungs, and muscles work together to help your body function best.

The purpose of this section is to help you understand the importance, benefits and methods of achieving fitness. This includes reasons why physical fitness is important following spinal cord injury (SCI), and ways to participate in fitness activities. This information is intended to be used with advice from your health care provider, physical therapist and/or occupational therapist to advance your exercise program.

Benefits of Exercise

Following SCI, many people become less active. Weight gain, loss of muscle tone and increased risk of cardiovascular disease can result. The activities of daily living or tasks of caring for your needs are not intense enough to provide cardiovascular fitness. Fitness can provide energy to actually perform the activities in your life. Physical wellness through aerobic and strengthening exercise may not be emphasized during the first few months after your injury. But, at the right time, your health care team can help you set up an appropriate exercise program.

Aerobic and strengthening exercises:
- Increase the heart's efficiency
- Increase blood flow to the lower extremities
- Increase your ability to perform activities of daily living
- Increase self-confidence
- Aid in a healthy body image
- Allow for social interaction
- Improve posture and postural pain
- Decrease risk of cardiovascular disease
- Reduce risk of overuse syndromes
- Aid in weight control
- Improve mood

Physical Fitness and Wellness Activities

Physical fitness and wellness after SCI can be achieved in many ways. Talk to your health care team about the best method. A beginning goal is to exercise at least three days a week and work up to at least five days a week.

Key points to remember:
- Start slow
- Establish a regular workout program
- Set goals
- Use the right equipment and dress appropriately
- Stay hydrated
- Pay attention to your body's signals
- Choose activities that fit your lifestyle and that you enjoy
- Stay committed

Aerobic Exercise

A good cardiovascular workout includes some sort of aerobic exercise. This type of exercise is continuous rhythmic movement that uses your body's major muscle groups and increases your heart rate. To benefit from aerobic exercise, you should move continuously for 20 to 30 minutes within your target heart rate range (see page 143 for more information), 3 to 5 times per week. Swimming and biking are examples of aerobic exercises. Your physical and occupational therapist can help you adapt to appropriate exercises.

These are other examples of aerobic exercise:
- Wheelchair biking
- Tai chi
- Pool aerobics or swimming
- Functional electrical stimulation (FES) leg biking (Figure 2)
- Seated wheelchair aerobic workout: Using upper arms and body, possibly with hand weights
- Upper arm ergometry: Similar to pedaling a bicycle with the arms

Other ways to get aerobic exercise comes from participation in adaptive sports such as basketball, rowing, biking, skiing, hockey or tennis. Adaptive equipment has been developed for almost every sport. Sports motivate people to continue exercise and many enjoy the competitive aspect.

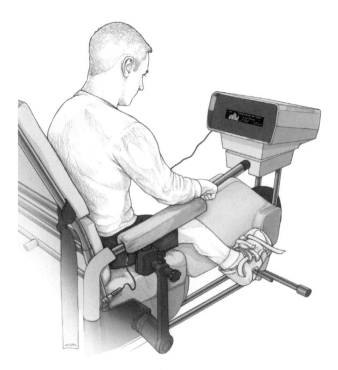

Figure 2. Functional electrical stimulation (FES) leg biking.

Strengthening Exercise

It is important to include strengthening exercises in your daily routine. Strong muscles improve posture, prevent injury and joint pain, and also can improve cardiovascular health. Strengthening activities may include weight lifting, Thera-Band® training, yoga, pilates, wheelchair push-ups, or other repetitive activities to strengthen muscle groups.

A weight lifting program should begin with lighter weights and focus on proper technique as indicated by your therapist or health care provider. When you have mastered proper technique, more weight can be added. To determine the appropriate weight that is safe for strengthening, work up to the weight at which your muscles fatigue after 10 to 15 repetitions. At this weight, perform an average of three sets of 10 repetitions. If you feel pain in any joint, decrease the amount of weight. If joint pain persists, you may need to adjust your technique. If you have questions regarding strengthening exercises, proper technique, or joint pain, talk to your physical or occupational therapist, health care provider, or certified fitness trainer.

Some additional examples of strengthening exercises are:

- Free weights
- Wall weights
- Exercise machines adapted for wheelchair users
- Resistance exercise bands (for example, Thera-Band®)
- Fitness ball workouts

Exercise Precautions

You should consult your health care team before beginning an exercise program. Blood pressure should be monitored before, during, and after exercise. High blood pressure during exercise can put abnormal stress on your cardiovascular system. To determine how hard you should exercise, find your target maximal heart rate. To do this, subtract your age from 220 to find your age-predicted maximal heart rate. The recommended exercise rate for individuals with SCI is 50 percent to 80 percent of their age-predicted maximal heart rate.

Individuals with SCI at or above the T6 level may have impaired control of their heart rate (pulse). Since the purpose of aerobic exercise is to elevate your heart rate, pulse monitoring may not be accurate. You must work with your health care team when starting an exercise program.

Skin protection should be considered during all activities. Skin on the areas listed below should be examined before and after a workout to check for pressure sore development:
- Elbow
- Shoulder blade
- Tailbone
- Side of hip
- Knee
- Ankle bone
- Heels

Look for areas of redness that do not resolve quickly, for blisters, openings in the skin, or rashes. You may need to alter your routine or add padding to equipment to eliminate future problems.

RELATIONSHIPS WITH FAMILIES AND LOVED ONES

You and your family may react to the changes caused by your spinal cord injury in different ways. You may think, "This can't be happening," or "You can't be serious, this has to be a mistake." It is normal for you and your family to experience a wide range of emotions after SCI.

This section provides information about the thoughts and feelings that are common following SCI, and may help you and your family to understand your reactions.

First Reactions, Concerns and Questions

A common first reaction to SCI is feeling grateful to be alive. However, this feeling is often accompanied by shock when you fully understand the seriousness of your injury. You and your family members may feel numb, confused, frightened and anxious. There may be uncertainty about what you are experiencing and what the future will bring. Such reactions are normal. Learning as much as possible about your injury can lessen everyone's confusion and anxiety. Understanding that your and your family's thoughts may range from denial to immediate recognition or acceptance following SCI is important.

Denial

You and your family may initially deny that your SCI is real and/or the seriousness of SCI. Denial is a normal way to cope with overwhelming feelings and can initially help prevent feelings of despair. However, denial can become a problem if reality is avoided for too long. You must move beyond denial to learn the information and skills necessary to adapt to the role SCI will play in everyone's life.

Recognition and acceptance

You and your family will eventually recognize that the injury has occurred, is long term and must be dealt with. Once you have moved past denial and experienced the grief associated with loss, you can start to cope with your injury and invest energy into regaining a positive quality of life.

Several things may influence your recognition and acceptance of SCI:
- *Cause of your injury:* Some individuals whose SCI was caused by a traumatic injury, such as a car accident, may not believe at first that they have a permanent injury. If your SCI is brought on slowly by disease of the spine, a gradual recognition may occur.

- *Alertness at the time of injury:* Those who are unconscious or under the influence of alcohol or drugs at the time of SCI may be less likely to recognize the permanence of their injury.
- *Pre-existing attitudes towards people with disabilities:* If you have had positive encounters with people who have disabilities in the past, you may accept your injury sooner. However, you may have believed that people with disabilities:
  — Should be pitied and given sympathy.
  — Should be praised because they are brave.
  — Should be avoided because they make others feel uncomfortable, anxious or afraid.
  — Have underlying emotional and thinking problems.
  — Are totally dependent on others.
  — Are second-class citizens, not entitled to the same rights and privileges of the nondisabled population.
  — Do not try hard enough to be independent.

If you have believed any of the above negative stereotypes concerning people with disabilities, you may be more reluctant to recognize your disability. It is important to recognize and deal with your own pre-existing beliefs. As a person with a disability, you should neither be praised nor pitied. Your accomplishments should be judged on the basis of your talents and limitations. Others may hold and apply the above-mentioned stereotypes to you. Therefore, you may be faced with educating family, friends and the nondisabled about living with a disability.

Emotions commonly experienced by you and your family

The feelings caused by a traumatic event such as SCI can be similar to those experienced when a family member dies. You may have preconceived ideas about what and how you are supposed to feel. These ideas may include the belief that you will go through specific stages in dealing with your injury. In reality, each person experiences and works through loss differently. As you begin to deal with what happened, you may experience some of the following feelings:

Why me?

You may ask, "Why me?" and similar questions when you are first injured. Although life is filled with unfair events, we rarely believe they will happen to us. Frequently the phrase "Why me?" is an expression of your anger or self-pity. This question has no satisfactory answer. The quicker you can refocus your thoughts on practical, solvable problems, the quicker the negative mood associated with "Why me?" will go away.

Grief and depression

Grief is defined as sad feelings related to a loss. These feelings are normal for you and your family members. During grief, self-esteem is usually not affected. Feelings of hopelessness or helplessness are usually absent, and you should respond positively to comfort and can still experience enjoyment.

Depression is defined as a sadness that is greater and more prolonged than what is expected. The term depression can imprecisely be used to describe everything from mild temporary sadness to suicidal hopelessness. However, the majority of people with SCI do not develop a true depressive disorder. It is important that if you have ongoing feelings of hopelessness and helplessness, or thoughts of ending your life, that you share these concerns with a member of your health care team.

Grief and depression have some aspects in common. Both can result in changes in sleep and appetite, along with painful and intense sadness. However, after SCI, changes in sleep and appetite may occur due to medical (pain) or hospital factors (being repositioned in bed throughout the night). These changes are not associated with depression.

Anger

You and your family may be angry about the onset or the cause of the injury. This anger may be directed toward your health care team members, the hospital or sometimes toward a higher being. You may also direct hostility and anger at your family members. Family members can be confused and hurt when greeted by angry outbursts. They need to understand that these outbursts are not usually personal attacks, but probably your frustration and anger about the injury.

At times, the anger of family members may be directed toward you or another person in the family. Explore these feelings with your family members before they become overwhelming. As a result, everyone may be able to communicate and cope more effectively. Writing a journal, recording your thoughts, or talking to someone outside of the situation (friend, minister, social worker or psychologist) are effective ways to deal with anger.

Spinal cord injury can make performing everyday activities slow, awkward and sometimes impossible. Activities usually require more planning and time. Demanding that things go smoothly can lead to frustration and anger.

To combat anger, it is important to recognize that:
- Pre-injury levels of speed and skill are not necessarily attainable
- The world will not end because your plans did not work out; it is only inconvenient
- Your frustration is not a catastrophe
- People in your life are doing the best they can

Guilt

If you caused your SCI, such as a car accident after drinking alcohol, you may feel guilty. This is a normal reaction. Remember that people are not perfect.

To reduce feelings of guilt, try to:
- Forgive yourself for your shortcomings, remind yourself that you are human
- Put the past behind you. Where needed, apologize to yourself or to others you offended
- Focus on improving your undesirable behaviors
- Remember your self-worth is distinct from your behavior
- Remember that others are responsible for their own feelings
- Share your feelings with others

Even if they had no role in causing your injury, family members may feel guilty, too. Phrases like, "I wish it had been me; you had so much life ahead of you," or "Why do I deserve to be walking around?" describe how many family members may feel. Feelings of guilt that are not understood or expressed can lead to overprotectiveness, misdirected anger, or in extreme cases, physical symptoms such as weight loss or gain, headaches, or upset stomach.

Anxiety

Anxiety is exaggerated or needless fear about possible negative events. Since most people know little about SCI and how to cope with it, anxiety is a natural reaction. You and your family members may be able to avoid or lessen anxiety by:
- Becoming fully informed about SCI
- Developing a trusting relationship with your health care team members
- Focusing your thoughts on events you can control
- Tracing your anxieties back to the thoughts and beliefs that caused them and replacing these thoughts or beliefs with more realistic ones
- Understanding that worrying about situations may make them worse, not better

- Using relaxation techniques to reduce tension, a product of anxiety
- Trying not to exaggerate the significance of things

Humor can also be an excellent way to reduce anxiety, and it can have mental and physical benefits. Humor is defined as perceiving what is amusing or comical. The ability to step back and not take the situation or yourself too seriously can help put things in perspective. Laughing can help make problems easier and increase positive mood. Those who have a sense of humor are frequently sought out by staff and other patients, thereby increasing social contact and support.

There are many ways to add humor to your life:
- Seek out funny friends and family
- Read comics in the daily newspaper
- Buy or borrow joke books
- Rent humorous videos or go see a comedy at the local theater
- Practice telling jokes to those you meet
- Watch comedies on television

Isolation
You and your family may feel abandoned or avoided following SCI. One reason could be others' shock and uncertainty about how to react and what to say to you. Rather than feeling like they are doing or saying the wrong things, those once close to you may pull away. Over time, some may return while others may not. To prevent isolating yourself from others, take the lead and re-establish social contacts.

Ways to handle uncomfortable situations without isolating yourself may include:
- *Family role playing:* You can invent problem social situations and act out responses that can be comfortably used by family members.
- *Confrontation:* Let others know how you feel when they do or say certain things. More honest communication should result.
- Explain your situation in simple terms.
- Ignore the situation.
- *Drop the "rejecters":* Seek out those you accept or who accept you. This is healthier than staying with people who are not understanding or supportive.

STRESS AND COPING SKILLS

Everyone experiences stress. Stress can be positive and encourage growth and opportunity, or it can be negative and may cause physical illness. Your reaction and how you manage stress determines whether it is positive or negative. Major life changes, such as spinal cord injury (SCI), can produce stress. When faced with SCI, your usual methods of coping may not work. Therefore, learning stress management and coping skills is important.

What is Stress?

Stress is defined as the body's response or reaction to physical and emotional demands. These demands can produce pleasure or pain. Stress can be beneficial. People often work best under moderate levels of stress. However, continuous stress may cause physical illness.

Stress triggers a physical reaction called the fight-or-flight response. This response prepares your body to either fight or flee from a threatening situation. When this happens, one or more of the following body functions may increase:
- Blood flow to muscles
- Blood pressure
- Breathing
- Heart rate
- Metabolism

What causes stress?

Events or situations that cause stress are called stressors. Negative stressors can be:
- *Physical:* Disease, traumatic injury
- *Environmental:* Climate, weather
- *Social:* Family illness, lack of support, conflict with others
- *Occupational:* Job loss, career change
- *Personal:* Not achieving your goals

Examples of positive stressors may include:
- A challenging job
- A wedding
- A birth in the family

Your reaction to an event or situation determines whether it is a negative or positive stressor.

What are the signs of stress?

Stress can cause physical, emotional and behavioral symptoms, such as:

Physical	Emotional	Behavorial
• Backaches	• Anger	• Absenteeism
• Headaches	• Depression	• Decreased concentration
• Fatigue	• Anxiety	• Emotional outbursts
• Insomnia	• Irritability	• Social withdrawal
• Frequent illness		• Tardiness
• Sexual difficulties		• Tearfulness
• Weight gain		• Increased smoking
• Weight loss		• Increased alcohol or drug use

How Can You Manage Stress?

Stress management refers to techniques that may help you deal with stress and reduce its harmful effects. The best stress management program is tailored to fit your needs. A tailored program requires you to carefully assess your experience with stress and describe current events or situations that are causing you stress. An effective stress management program includes a plan for a healthy lifestyle, such as regular exercise, good nutrition and preventive medical care.

Focus on the way you think

Change how you think about a situation, event or stressor that triggers a negative stress response. When you have a negative thought, try to make it positive. For example, if you can't do some things that you did before your injury, don't focus on what you can't do. Instead, reframe your thought to, "This is an opportunity for me to try some new things."

Keep things in perspective and maintain a positive attitude. Many of us worry about things that will never happen, or that we cannot control. While it is hard to be happy all the time, focus on the positive and don't waste your energy worrying about things you have no control over.

Relaxation skills

Learning to relax your body (opposite of the fight-or-flight response) is important. Several relaxation techniques include visual or guided imagery, muscle relaxation and relaxed breathing. Caffeine and nicotine can interfere with relaxation. Therefore, it is important to avoid using them for at least one hour before practicing relaxation techniques.

Visual or guided imagery

Guidelines for visual or guided imagery include:

- Get comfortable in your chair or bed.
- Close your eyes and concentrate on your breathing.
- Relax your body, letting the chair or bed support you completely.
- Picture in your mind a relaxing, pleasant scene, such as lying on a beach on a warm day or looking down from a mountaintop.
- Focus your mind on that scene. Picture yourself in the scene and focus on sights, smells and sensations.
- Continue to picture this scene for 10 to 20 minutes. Slowly open your eyes and focus on your surroundings.

Muscle relaxation

Two techniques for relaxing your muscles include autogenic relaxation and progressive muscle relaxation. Autogenic means that this technique comes from your thoughts. Most individuals with SCI can learn autogenic relaxation. Your ability to perform progressive muscle relaxation will depend on the level of your SCI, as it involves physically tensing and relaxing muscles.

Guidelines for autogenic relaxation exercise include:

- Perform the exercise at least two times per day.
- Do the exercise where you are free from interruption or outside stimulation.
- Choose a focus word, phrase or image that you find relaxing.
- Sit or lie in a comfortable position.
- Close your eyes.
- Relax your muscles as you are able.
- Breathe slowly and naturally, focusing on your chosen word, phrase or image.
- Continue to relax for 10 to 20 minutes. If your mind wanders, concentrate on your breathing and your focus word, phrase or image again.
- When you are finished, remain quiet for a few minutes, first with your eyes closed, then open.

Guidelines for progressive muscle relaxation exercise include:

- Perform the exercise once or twice each day.
- Do the exercise for 20 to 30 minutes each time.
- Choose a place where you are free from interruption or outside stimulation.
- If you wish, remove glasses or contact lenses.
- Concentrate on relaxed breathing for at least two minutes before you begin.

- Tense each of the following muscle groups as you are able, for at least five seconds and then relax for at least 30 seconds. Focus your attention on the sensations of tension and relaxation and the difference between the two. Repeat before moving to the next muscle group.
  — *Upper part of face:* Lift eyebrows toward ceiling, feeling tension in your forehead and scalp.
  — *Central part of face:* Squint eyes tightly, wrinkle nose and mouth, feeling tension in the middle part of your face.
  — *Lower part of face:* Clench your teeth and pull the corners of your mouth back towards your ears. Feel the tension in your mouth and jaw.
  — *Neck:* Gently touch your chin to your chest. Feel the pull in the back of your neck spread into your head.
  — *Shoulders:* Pull your shoulders up toward your ears. Feel the tension in your shoulders, head, neck and down your back.
  — *Upper arms:* Pull your arms back and press your elbows toward the sides of your body. Try not to tense your forearms. Feel the tension in your arms, shoulders and into your back.
  — *Hands and lower arms:* Make a tight fist and pull up your wrists. Feel the tension in your hand, knuckles and up into the forearm.
  — *Chest, shoulders and upper back:* Pull back your shoulders as if you are trying to make your shoulder blades touch.
  — *Stomach:* Pull your stomach toward your spine.
  — *Upper legs:* Squeeze your knees together and lift your legs off the chair or bed. Feel the tension in your thighs.
  — *Lower legs:* Raise your feet toward the ceiling while flexing your feet toward your body. Feel the tension in your calf area.
  — *Feet:* Turn your feet inward and curl your toes up and out.

Relaxed breathing

The goals of relaxed breathing are to slow your breathing and to reduce the use of shoulder, neck and upper chest muscles, allowing you to breathe more efficiently. You can use relaxed breathing anytime — before and during stressful situations or to relieve shortness of breath.

The following guidelines help you practice relaxed breathing:
- Sit or lie in a comfortable position.
- Loosen any tight clothing around your abdomen and waist.
- Rest your hands in your lap or at your side.

- Breathe in slowly and deeply through your nose (if possible). Allow your abdomen to expand as you breathe in.
- Exhale at your normal rate.

If you cannot feel your abdomen expand as you breathe in:
- As you breathe out, gently push against your abdomen with your hand.
- Breathe in, allowing your abdomen to expand against your hand.

Practice relaxed breathing throughout the day until it becomes natural for you. Use this technique even when you are not anxious or stressed.

Coping Skills

Coping skills are important in learning to deal with your surroundings and social situations both in and out of the hospital. Each person has their own way of responding to lifestyle changes. These include thoughts, feelings and actions. You may need to develop and rely on new coping strategies after your SCI.

Coping Skills While in the Hospital

You can begin to use coping skills while in the hospital, during recovery and rehabilitation. Helpful coping skills include gathering information, finding social support, communicating openly, being assertive and getting away from the hospital.

Gathering information

Gather and read as much information about your condition as possible, to help you better understand your injury. Talk to members of your health care team about the level and completeness of your SCI, which determines the body functions that are affected. You may also want to see visual images of your spine or spinal cord to understand the location and extent of your injury.

Peer mentors are another resource for information. Peer mentors are individuals who also have SCI and talk to others about living with the condition, ways to cope and services available in the community. If your SCI is recent, you may initially feel uncomfortable talking to a peer mentor. However, a visit can be helpful and informative. If you are interested in meeting with a peer mentor, ask a member of your health care team to arrange a visit.

Social support

Social support from family, friends and staff can make you feel cared for and is important. Those with a recent SCI are frequently surprised by how many people write or visit. This social support can help reduce negative emotions such as anger and anxiety, build self-esteem and increase openness to new information. The crisis of an SCI presents an opportunity to renew and to strengthen personal relationships. Actively encourage friends and family to write, call and visit. Let them know that you appreciate their concern.

Open communication

The ability to openly communicate your feelings and beliefs is important. Discussing your feelings is usually easiest with those you trust. Yet sometimes these individuals are the hardest to talk with. This may be due to your loved one's need to protect you or pretend that he or she is happy. You cannot be responsible for another person's feelings. An open and honest sharing of concerns and feelings will lead to better communication and to a greater sense of mutual support.

Being assertive

SCI may force people who were physically independent to depend on others. Communicating your needs and desires assertively is crucial to successfully coping with SCI. Express your thoughts and feelings honestly and directly. Being assertive involves respecting yourself and others at the same time. By letting people know your desires, you may be in a better position to have them fulfilled, which can help you feel in control.

Coping Skills After Leaving the Hospital

While in the rehabilitation unit, it may be easy to push your wheelchair. Bathrooms are accessible and people don't stare at you with puzzled looks. After being discharged from the hospital, you face a world of steps, uneven surfaces, inaccessible bathrooms, unreliable transportation and uninformed people.

After leaving the hospital rehabilitation unit, you may still need time to adapt to your new lifestyle and evaluate your physical and personal situation. This process may take longer than you think and should be gradual. At first, you may want to enter places with the fewest architectural and social barriers. Then, move on to more challenging settings. Coping outside the rehabilitation unit will require learning skills such as setting new goals, developing a social support network, finding a meaningful lifestyle and remembering you are a unique person.

Set new goals

SCI requires a new lifestyle. To cope with this change, you must be flexible and experiment with new ways to achieve your goals. Part of your long-term adjustment to SCI will be to set new goals and develop new interests. Even though you have a disability, being active tends to make you healthier and happier.

Think about the future. Plan to return to employment. See the section *Going Back to Work*, Chapter Eight, for more information. If you cannot return to your previous job, consider training for a new position or going back to school. Set both short-term (within one year) and long-term (one to five years) goals. Never forget that for each thing you can no longer do, there are many others that you can. Focus on what you can do. Many people with SCI invent remarkable solutions to problems.

Develop a social support network

Develop supportive relationships that reduce the effects of social isolation and improve the quality of your life. Developing a social network can begin by working on your communication skills and joining a support or mutual interest group. Today there are many opportunities on the Internet to join chat rooms, blogs or similar mediums to share concerns, get new ideas, and learn more about day-to-day challenges and solutions to living with SCI.

Find a meaningful lifestyle

Although new interests may develop following SCI, most likely your pre-injury interests will not change. However, you may experience physical problems acting on your interests, such as performing a physically demanding job, hobby or sport. Many jobs and activities are still possible, but may require a different way of doing them.

Your biggest challenge is returning to a productive, meaningful lifestyle. Many people think a productive lifestyle means returning to paid employment. However, your "new" productive lifestyle may or may not include this. What matters is using your time meaningfully. Participate in activities you like. Use your abilities and talents to contribute to your community. Plan a productive nonwork life-style. The more positive your approach, the more you will get out of life. Consider joining groups, such as wheelchair sports, social action groups, nature groups—whatever fits your interests.

Remember you are a unique person

An SCI can negatively impact your sense of self-worth. Activities that once brought a sense of accomplishment may now be difficult or impossible. Self-care activities may have to be relearned using special equipment. However, your worth as a person does not depend on your accomplishments. You are still the same unique and worthwhile person. Take pride in the unique qualities that make you who you are. Your sense of pride and self-worth influences how you dress, talk and behave.

Things you can do to increase your self-worth include:
- Set attainable rehabilitation goals, both physical and mental. Keep track of your progress in attaining your goals
- List your unique qualities. Think of ways to express these qualities despite your disability
- Take pride in your appearance

Integration into the Community

Stereotypes

You may find that public attitudes can make the move back into the community difficult. The general public sometimes views people with disabilities as if they:
- Should be pitied
- Require constant care
- Should be segregated from society
- Would not make good friends
- Are difficult to communicate with
- Are emotionally unstable

Nondisabled people often have false ideas or stereotypes about people with a disability because of:
- Ignorance
- Anxiety that a similar disability could happen to them
- Fear of embarrassing or offending the disabled person
- Linking impaired physical function to general impairment as a person
- Assuming the disability reflects punishment for misdeeds

The public can apply inappropriate positive labels to the disabled, too. They can falsely view the disabled as more intelligent, adjusted and considerate.

Social Skills Needed for Success

Generally, society expects nondisabled people to be kind and helpful toward those who have a disability. This may make nondisabled people feel uneasy. As a result, both disabled and nondisabled people may not truthfully say or do what they are thinking or feeling. This can further complicate social interactions. Developing and practicing social skills may help to reduce strained interactions.

Social skills needed for successful integration include:
- General social skills
- General disability social skills
- SCI-specific social skills

General social skills

General social skills lead to effective and rewarding communication and are important to the disabled and nondisabled. General social skills include:
- Listening
- Receiving compliments gracefully
- Starting a conversation
- Maintaining a conversation
- Assertiveness
- Confrontation
- Appropriate self-disclosure
- Using humor effectively
- Appropriate touch
- Maintaining appropriate eye contact

Most people practice these social skills. However, they become more important for someone with a physical disability. You are likely to have more positive interactions if you use humor to decrease the anxiety felt by the nondisabled and appropriately assert yourself.

General disability social skills

General disability social skills are helpful if you have an obvious disability. Negative stereotypes held by the general public may lead them to behave inappropriately. For example, when a wheelchair user appears to be struggling with a barrier, nondisabled people may, without asking permission, forcefully grab the wheelchair in an attempt to be helpful. This awkward social situation may require special skills unique to using a wheelchair. Some examples of situations and social skills you could use are illustrated in the following table.

Situation	What to do
• Undesired help is offered	• Refuse help gracefully and thank the person
• Undesired social advances	• Assertively tell the person that you prefer to be left alone
• Staring	• Ignore it, or smile
• Unwanted questions	• Gently say, "I'd rather not talk about that."
• Someone displays a lack of knowledge about your disability	• Honestly tell that person about your disability
• You need help	• Ask for help

SCI-specific social skills

Some social skills are unique to SCI, such as managing bowel and bladder accidents, or handling reactions to deformities or disfigurement. Change in appearance of hands or legs, or the use of prostheses (artificial body parts) may evoke unwanted reactions from the nondisabled. Social situations will go smoother if appropriate social skills and reactions (examples noted in above table) can be practiced in advance and used when needed.

SUBSTANCE ABUSE AND ADDICTION

Chemical health is the process of choosing environments, engaging in behaviors and making decisions that reduce or eliminate the problematic use of chemicals such as alcohol, nicotine, caffeine, prescription and non-prescription medications, and illegal drugs. For clarity, these chemicals are referred to as "substances." Choosing to be chemically healthy is especially important following spinal cord injury (SCI), since some of your body functions have changed. The use and misuse of mood-altering or addictive substances can lead to substance abuse, addiction and physical consequences.

When Does Use Become Addiction or Abuse?

A blanket definition of misuse or abuse of substances is difficult because each person's situation is unique. Addiction is a chronic disease characterized by:

- Using the substance regularly and/or excessively
- Spending a great deal of time thinking about getting and using the substance
- Denying a problem with substance use
- Hiding the substance, using the substance alone, or being secretive about your use
- Inability to stop using or reduce your use of the substance for long periods
- Doing things to get the substance that you normally would not do (for example, stealing or lying)
- Using the substance to escape from problems
- Driving or doing other activities that place you and others at risk when under the influence of the substance
- Using an illegal substance
- Using medication more often, in larger doses, or for purposes other than prescribed or recommended
- Using alcohol or other substances with medication

Even if you aren't addicted, a substance can still cause problems. This is referred to as substance abuse. Substance abuse is repeatedly using too much of a substance, such as alcohol, and that use leads to health or other problems. Unlike those who are addicted, people who abuse a substance are not physically dependent on it.

Statistics show that a large percentage of traumatic spinal cord injuries are substance related, particularly motor vehicle crashes while driving under the influence of alcohol. If alcohol use was a problem for you before your SCI, likely, the problem will continue. Therefore, it is important to understand how substance use can affect your body and mind following SCI.

Physical and Psychological Effects

Everyone needs to be aware of the effects of substances such as alcohol, nicotine, caffeine, prescription and non-prescription medications, and illegal drugs. However, these substances can affect you even more after SCI and may interfere with prescribed medications by increasing their potency or decreasing their effectiveness.

The following list describes how substances can affect your thinking, mood and behavior following SCI.
- Difficulty concentrating
- Difficulty learning
- Memory loss
- Impaired reasoning, planning and judgment

- Distorted perception of reality (what is actually real and what is not)
- Tendency to deny the severity of your injury
- Depression
- Decreased self-esteem
- Agitation
- Sluggishness (lethargy)
- Lack of motivation to achieve goals
- Inability to deal with your loss through the grieving process
- Social inhibition
- Increased thoughts of self-harm

Many of these behaviors, changes in mood and thinking can affect your physical health, as indicated on the following pages.

Alcohol

All alcoholic beverages contain the drug ethanol. The amount of ethanol in your blood is called blood alcohol level. The effects of alcohol are related to how much is in your blood. The more alcohol in the blood, the greater its effect on your thinking, mood, behavior and body. Blood alcohol level is determined by how quickly you drink and how fast your body can break down (metabolize) the alcohol.

After SCI, you lose weight because you lose muscle mass. In addition, the lack of activity in your paralyzed muscles leads to a slower rate of alcohol metabolism. With the combination of reduced weight and a lower metabolic rate, the same amount of alcohol you drank before your injury will result in a higher blood alcohol level after your injury. The alcohol's effect may also remain longer than before your injury. If you continue to use alcohol, you should be careful to do so in moderation, since the effect may be different now. Moderate alcohol use is no more than two servings of alcohol every 24 hours. A serving of alcohol is one 12 oz. can of beer, one 4 oz. glass of wine, or 1 oz. of hard liquor.

The psychological affects of alcohol, such as impaired reasoning, planning and judgment, can cause further injuries due to increased risk of accidents, burns and falls. The increase in fluid consumption and impaired thinking can disrupt your catheterization schedule. Overfilling your bladder can cause it to stretch or may weaken the muscle lining. This may cause fluid to flow back into the kidneys, increasing your risk for bladder or kidney infection, autonomic hyperreflexia (dysreflexia) and urinary incontinence (accidents).

Effects of alcohol can also damage your skin. Urinary or bowel incontinence causes excessive moisture to the skin. Alcohol can lead to poor nutrition and dehydration, increasing the risk for skin breakdown and decreasing your body's ability to heal itself. Impaired thinking can also lead you to neglect weight shifts and be careless with transfers. Both of these can cause injury to your skin.

Nicotine

Nicotine is a highly addictive substance found in tobacco products such as cigarettes, cigars and chewing tobacco. Nicotine has a powerful effect on the body, changing mood, alertness and energy levels. These effects are pleasing and, therefore, reinforce tobacco use. Over time, your body adapts to an expected level of nicotine in the system, and a "normal" state is achieved only when smoking or using chewing tobacco routinely.

Heart disease (also referred to as coronary artery disease) is the most common cause of death among Americans. The relationship between cigarette smoking and coronary artery disease has been well known for years. SCI impairs the muscles involved in breathing and, therefore, smoking places you at additional risk for injury to your lungs. Smoking causes an increased buildup of secretions in your lungs that are difficult to expel due to muscle weakness. This results in a higher risk of pneumonia and atelectasis (collapsed lung).

Smoking also decreases the amount of oxygen in the bloodstream needed to nourish tissues and muscles. This can lead to increased incidence of skin breakdown and a reduced ability to heal not only skin, but bones as well. Smoking is also known to worsen neuropathic pain (sharp, shooting or burning pain at or below the level of injury).

Chewing tobacco does not affect the lungs, but can cause serious diseases in the mouth, throat and stomach. Because of the amount of nicotine delivered through chewing tobacco, the heart rate and blood pressure changes which occur when chewing are similar to those experienced by smokers. Additional health problems can include gum recession, tooth decay, tooth loss, ulcer formation, and cancer of the mouth, throat and esophagus.

Shortly after stopping nicotine use, you may feel uncomfortable and abnormal. Withdrawal symptoms begin within hours of the last use, as nicotine levels in the body drop. Symptoms may include irritability, anxiety, frustration, inability to concentrate, decreased heart rate and insomnia. Despite potential withdrawal symptoms, stopping nicotine use has major and immediate health benefits. Talk to your health care provider for information about nicotine replacement therapy, counseling, quitlines and other support methods to help you stop using nicotine.

Caffeine

Caffeine is a naturally occurring substance found in certain plants, for example, cocoa beans or tea leaves. Beverages that contain caffeine such as coffee, tea or soft drinks, have a diuretic effect. This means that after you drink them, your body loses water through increased urination. The more caffeine consumed, the greater potential for increased fluid loss and perhaps dehydration.

For persons with SCI, caffeine consumption can increase urine volume in your bladder, stretching the bladder or increasing bladder pressure. This places you at risk for kidney problems. Too much caffeine intake may cause jitters, anxiety and insomnia, may temporarily speed up your heart rate, and can trigger autonomic hyperreflexia.

Talk to your health care provider about how much caffeine is appropriate for you. If you consume too much caffeine, develop a caffeine reduction plan and cut back gradually.

Prescription and non-prescription medications

Your health care provider may prescribe different medications following SCI. Sedatives (to relieve anxiety or insomnia) and narcotic medications (to relieve pain) can be particularly habit-forming. Most people who take medication as directed—the correct amount for the prescribed time as determined by your health care provider—do not become addicted. However, serious problems sometimes develop if medications are misused. Taking a pain or non-prescription medication for purposes other than pain relief, or not taking a medication as prescribed, can be considered misuse. Persons who have had a history of substance abuse or dependence are at greater risk of abuse or dependence on prescription drugs.

Narcotic medications depress the functioning of the central nervous system. This can lead to impaired judgment, reduced muscular coordination, drowsiness, and risk for accidents and falls. Narcotics can also slow bowel function, causing constipation or stool impaction. When used with alcohol, narcotic medications can cause respiratory failure and death.

If you begin to take medication more often, in larger doses, or for purposes other than those prescribed or recommended, or if you feel the need to add other substances to achieve the desired effect, talk with your health care provider. You should honestly and openly discuss any past history of medication abuse with current or future health care providers.

Illegal drugs

Illegal drugs include any type of controlled substance not prescribed by a physician, such as:

- *Cannabis:* Marijuana and hashish
- *Central nervous system stimulants:* Amphetamines, methamphetamines and cocaine
- *Hallucinogens:* LSD, mushrooms and PCP
- *Opioids and opiates:* Heroin, morphine, codeine and methadone
- *Other substances:* Synthetic compounds (Ecstasy) and inhalants (glue, paint, solvents and nitrous oxide)

Misuse of such drugs can lead to heart, lung and brain damage, depression, insomnia and memory loss. It is widely accepted that illegal drugs do not have any therapeutic value if not prescribed by a physician and they can be especially dangerous if you have SCI. Long-term use of stimulants can decrease appetite, causing weight loss and increasing your risk for pressure ulcers or skin breakdown. Also, stimulants cause blood pressure to rise, increasing the risk associated with autonomic hyperreflexia.

Assessing Your Drug Use

Assessing your past alcohol or drug use is the first step in changing use patterns. A diagnosis of addiction usually requires assessment by a psychiatrist, psychologist or a specialized addiction counselor. However, answering the following questions (referred to as the CAGE Assessment) can help you determine if follow-up with a mental health specialist is needed. This assessment may also help you plan how alcohol or drug use may or may not fit into your lifestyle following SCI.

CAGE Assessment

- Have you ever felt you should **C**ut down on your alcohol or drug use?
- Have people **A**nnoyed you by criticizing your alcohol or drug use?
- Have you ever felt bad or **G**uilty about your alcohol or drug use?
- Have you ever used alcohol or drugs first thing in the morning (as an "**E**ye-opener") to steady your nerves or get rid of a hangover?

If you answered "yes" to any question, you should talk to your health care provider about whether you have a chemical health problem.

Treatment

Change in your substance use begins with admitting that you have a chemical health problem and assessing your motivation to change your behavior. This includes asking yourself the following questions:

- How motivated am I to change my substance use?
- How confident am I in my ability to change my substance use?

Answering these questions can help you assess whether you are ready and willing to seek help for your substance use.

Research has significantly increased what is known about treatment for the different types of substance use. Various treatments are available, such as Alcoholics Anonymous (AA) or nicotine cessation centers. Consult your health care provider to discuss treatment options and determine which plan best fits your situation.

This plan may include:

- Limiting occasions where you use substances, as well as setting boundaries with family and friends you have used substances with in the past.
- Practicing refusal statements such as, "My health care provider said absolutely no alcohol with the medications I am on," or "No thanks, I've stopped smoking since my accident." Your SCI provides you with a socially acceptable reason to change your substance use.
- Attending only those activities that do not involve substances.

Coping Strategies for Family Members

Living with someone who abuses or is addicted to substances can be extremely difficult. If someone in your family has a substance abuse or addiction problem, these tips may help:

- *Attend a support group:* These groups provide encouragement and information about your family member's condition and insight into how substance misuse affects the entire family. Support groups for family members may include Alcoholics Anonymous, Al-Anon and Nar-Anon (for adults affected by someone else's substance abuse) and Alateen (for teenage children whose parents have a substance use problem). To locate a support group in your community, talk with your health care provider or check the phone book, local newspaper, or the Internet.

- *Learn as much as possible about substance abuse and addiction:* Some of your behaviors and beliefs may inadvertently contribute to substance use, such as the belief that drinking alcohol regularly is harmless. Ignore comments from those who suggest that using substances is an understandable and acceptable way of coping with SCI. Such comments are inappropriate and potentially harmful.

- *Be patient and supportive:* Recovery takes time. Express pride in your family member's efforts to overcome a substance problem. The focus should be on the individual who has a problem and not on substance abuse issues.

- *Encourage communication:* Listen carefully while your family member expresses feelings. Respond without placing guilt or blame.

- If you think the addiction is life threatening, seek emergency help immediately.

Resources

Chemical health support groups such as local AA chapters or nicotine quit lines are available to assist in the recovery process. Talk to your health care provider about additional resources.

AGING

Life expectancy for persons with spinal cord injury has increased almost to a normal life span. Aging changes everyone's bodies and organ systems. Some changes may be accelerated or require more attention for those who have SCI. Understanding these changes can help prevent secondary complications and maintain your level of functional independence.

Aging affects organ systems as well as your ability to perform tasks of daily living. Though everyone ages differently, aging-related changes affect your skin, muscles and bones, as well as the digestive, urinary and nervous systems. A person with an SCI must be aware of additional concerns, besides just getting older. Knowing these SCI-related problems and practicing healthy living behaviors are important.

Basic Preventive Care

Basic preventive care includes a healthy diet, fitness, safety precautions, close skin inspection and regular screening tests. Standard screening tests and immunizations are important after SCI. Your injury may require more frequent visits to the doctor than normally recommended (Table 2).

Skin

Aging skin loses elasticity. Drooping or wrinkling can occur not only on the face, but also the buttocks, abdomen, arms and legs. The skin also becomes thinner, so veins or discolorations beneath the surface are more visible than when you were younger. Decreased production of natural oils may dry out the skin and lessen perspiration. Loose, thin and dry skin injures more easily and can take longer to heal than young, healthy skin.

After SCI, monitoring and caring for aging skin are especially important. Those with SCI are more prone to develop pressure sores, blisters, cracks, tears or shearing. Your weight and posture may also change, altering the pressure distribution on skin (especially in the back, buttocks, and upper legs) when sitting for long periods. You may need to turn or adjust positions in your chair more often. The ability to perform transfers may also change. Poor transfers can lead to friction, shear (when skin moves in one direction and the underlying bone moves in another) or skin tears. Transfers, seating system and cushions should be evaluated yearly to assure adequate transfers and pressure relief.

Moisture from perspiration, urine or stool can also cause skin breakdown. Effective bowel and bladder management are important. Avoid nylon undergarments, which hold moisture, and try not to allow large creases of hems under your buttocks or legs. Avoid homemade covers for your wheelchair cushion. They can lead to high-pressure areas. Do not use inflatable "donut" type cushions, which can cause increased pressure to the skin inside the "donut" edges. If you are hospitalized, review your skin management program with the staff so they can continue your program, as you direct, to avoid skin breakdown.

Sun protection

Over time, the sun's ultraviolet (UV) light damages skin. UV radiation from the sun is the main cause of skin cancer. Protecting your

Table 2 Recommended preventive screenings and immunizations

	Non-Injured Male	Non-Injured Female	Persons with SCI
Weight	Annually	Annually	Annually
Blood pressure	Every 2 years	Every 2 years	Every 2 years*
Blood cholesterol	Every 5 years after age 40	Every 5 years after age 40	Annually
Colon	Every 5 to 10 years after age 50	Every 5 to 10 years after age 50	Every 5 to 10 years after age 50, unless change in bowel pattern
Blood sugar	Every 3 years after age 45	Every 3 years after age 45	Annually
Skin examination	Every 2 to 3 years after age 40 for a skin cancer check	Every 2 to 3 years after age 40 for a skin cancer check	Daily self-skin examination for pressure sores; every 2 to 3 years after age 40 for a skin cancer check
Prostate	PSA (prostate-specific antigen) test and digital rectal examination yearly after age 50	N/A	PSA (prostate-specific antigen) test and digital rectal examination yearly for males after age 50
Breast	N/A	Annual mammogram after age 40	Annual mammogram for females after age 40
Bone density	N/A	Baseline at menopause	3 to 5 years after SCI for both males and females, and age 30 for baseline; one year later to check for bone loss and again after limb fracture or change in mobility (or after menopause for females and after age 55 for males)
Influenza immunization	Annually after age 50 if you have chronic disease, or contact with high-risk people	Annually after age 50 if you have chronic disease, or contact with high-risk people	Annually
Pneumonia vaccine (one lifetime dose but may need second dose if high risk)	Age 65 or older, or if you have a medical condition that increases risk	Age 65 or older, or if you have a medical condition that increases risk	Initial dose soon after injury; may need repeat dose after 5 years
Zostavax (Shingles vaccine)	Age 60 or older, or age 50 or older if you have a medical condition that increases risk	Age 60 or older, or age 50 or older if you have a medical condition that increases risk	One-time dose soon after injury

*Blood pressure should be checked every visit for a person with an injury above T6 or at anytime a person with autonomic hyperreflexia has symptoms of it.

skin by minimizing direct exposure to sunlight and by using sun screen daily, is important.

Tips for preventing skin problems include:
- Good nutrition and hydration
- Healthy body weight
- Appropriate equipment for transfers
- Twice daily skin checks
- Good bowel and bladder care to avoid incontinence (accidents)
- Frequent position changes in bed and in your wheelchair
- Yearly evaluation of your seating system
- Skin protection from sun exposure
- No tobacco use
- Prompt treatment if pressure ulcers (open sores caused by prolonged pressure) arise

Muscles, Bones and Joints

Muscles

With aging, muscles lose strength and flexibility. Reflexes tend to slow, and balance and coordination can decline. You may feel more fatigued due to increased weakness and the effort it takes to accomplish certain activities. Therefore, you may need more adaptive equipment, time or assistance to achieve activities. Generally mild muscle changes are expected with aging. However, you may need to be more vigilant with a strengthening and exercise program. New or increased weakness should be evaluated by your health care provider.

To prevent muscle problems:
- Maintain a regular stretching program and physical activity as you are able.
- Consume a balanced diet.
- Conserve energy by resting between activities, or organizing tasks to prevent or minimize fatigue.
- Prioritize activities.
- Use adaptive equipment.

Bones

Rather than being hard, rigid and unchanging, bones constantly undergo renewal and respond to the demands placed on them. Bones reach their maximal mass between ages 25 to 35. Then, they decline slightly in size and density. As they change, bones become more brittle and prone to fractures.

Osteoperosis

Osteoporosis is a condition caused by a gradual loss of minerals (such as calcium and phosphorous) from bones. Mineral loss leaves bones thinner, weaker and more prone to fracture. Bone mass loss begins after age 30 and increases in postmenopausal women. Bone loss happens more quickly in men and women with SCI due to the lack of weight-bearing stress on the skeleton. This loss begins within days of your injury and continues for months to years, below the level of injury.

Unlike other bone and joint problems, osteoporosis begins without physical symptoms. A bone fracture may be the first indication. Fractures occur more commonly in persons with SCI in the lower extremities, typically from falls or other injuries. The fracture usually presents as swelling, rather than pain, and possible increased spasticity (involuntary tightening or movement of the muscles) or autonomic hyperreflexia (dysreflexia).

To help prevent bone problems:
- Maintain the activity level prescribed by your health care provider or therapist.
- Utilize functional electrical stimulation (FES), a technique that uses electrical currents to stimulate the nerves affected by paralysis. Sometimes FES includes neuroprostheses (an artificial device used to replace or improve the function of an impaired nervous system), which allow people with paraplegia to walk, those with quadriplegia to stand and/or have restored hand-grasp function, and increased bowel and bladder function. Ask your health care provider if FES would be beneficial.
- Strengthen bones by standing. If you cannot stand on your own, a standing frame may be beneficial in preventing osteoporosis.
- Maintain calcium in your diet. Talk to your health care provider regarding a supplement if your diet does not supply sufficient calcium.
- Take medication (biphosphonates) if prescribed by your health care provider. Bisphosphonates decrease the rate of bone loss, increase bone mineral density and decrease risk of fracture. Examples include Fosamax™ (Alendronate), Boniva™ (ibandronate) and Actonel™ (risedronate).

Joints

Arthritis

Arthritis is inflammation and wear-and-tear of a joint, leading to deterioration. Heredity, diet, being overweight, previous injuries and diseases in the joints are possible contributors. However, so is everyday use.

Osteoarthritis

Osteoarthritis, sometimes called degenerative arthritis or degenerative joint disease, causes pain and stiffness and starts in the spine or large joints (such as the hips or knees). Because a natural response to a painful joint is to move it less, you may also decrease muscle use in the area of pain, causing muscles to shrink and lose strength.

Overuse syndromes

Overuse syndromes occur when joints and muscles repeatedly do tasks that they were not designed to do, such as propelling a manual wheelchair, transferring from one surface to another, or walking with crutches or a walker. Any joint can be affected by overuse, causing pain, increased muscle tone, numbness and tingling, and poor posture. These syndromes often develop in the upper extremities, but also can develop in the lower extremities. Most common overuse syndromes involve the shoulder and elbow, with pain occurring during use. However, other conditions such as carpal tunnel syndrome can also occur. These injuries can occur soon after SCI, but become more common with aging.

To help prevent joint problems:
- Try to avoid repetitive motion.
- Use push gloves to propel a manual wheelchair.
- Explore equipment options such as a power assist or a power wheelchair.
- Include padded handgrips on canes or crutches.
- Modify transfer techniques.
- Evaluate adaptive equipment for the home and work space.
- Allow for rest periods and limit use of the muscle and joint if symptoms develop.

Heart and Circulatory System

Even a healthy heart changes with age. Your heart muscle becomes less elastic and a less efficient pump and must work harder to do the same job. Your heart is strong enough to meet the body's normal needs. However, it has less reserve capacity for overcoming injury or handling the sudden demands from stress or illness.

Cardiovascular disease is the leading cause of mortality among men and women in the general population. Cardiovascular disease is associated with high risk of heart attack, stroke and other complications. People with SCI tend to have an earlier onset of cardiovascular disease. Physical inactivity and weight gain decrease muscle and lean body mass, increasing the percentage of body fat and the risk for cardiovascular disease and diabetes in persons who have SCI.

To help prevent heart and circulatory system problems:
- Monitor your blood cholesterol and blood pressure.
- Maintain a healthy weight.
- Pay attention to dietary factors.
- Reduce saturated fats, trans fats and cholesterol in your diet.
  — Saturated fats are found mainly in animal products, including whole milk, cheese, butter, beef, pork, lamb, as well as palm oil, coconut oil, cocoa butter and hydrogenated oils.
  — Trans fats should be avoided. These fats are found in baked goods, processed foods, some margarines, shortening and some forms of peanut butter.
  — Moderate consumption of monosaturated fats, with no more than 30 percent of calories coming from fat. Monosaturated fats help lower blood cholesterol levels if eaten in limited amounts. They can be found in olive, peanut and canola oil.
  — Limit consumption of sodium. Sodium attracts and holds water in the body and excess fluid retention can put added stress on the heart and blood vessels to pump the extra fluid. The recommendation by the American Heart Association is 2,000 mg to 3,000 mg per day. Foods to limit include pre-packaged items, fast food, canned soups and vegetables, deli meats, cheese, snack foods and condiments (soy sauce, ketchup, salad dressing).
  – Increase soluble fiber intake to help lower cholesterol. Soluble fiber is found in citrus fruits, strawberries, apples, legumes, oatmeal and oat bran, or as a supplement. Insoluble fiber stimulates the GI tract and is found in foods such as vegetables, wheat bran and whole wheat grain breads. The recommended amount to consume is 10 grams to 25 grams per day of soluble fiber and at least 25 grams to 30 grams of total fiber per day.
  — Increase consumption of sterols or stanols, which have been found to reduce LDL cholesterol levels. Examples of products that contain sterols or stanols are Benecol™ and Take Control™. Recommended levels are 2 grams per day, every day. Typically, results can be seen after two weeks of correct use.

— Consume omega 3 fatty acids, which help prevent cardio-vascular disease. The American Heart Association recommends 1 gram of omega 3 fatty acids per day. Good sources are fish and fish oils. At least two servings of fish are recommended per week.
— Don't drink. However, if you do, limit alcohol intake, since 1 to 2 servings per day may reduce cardiovascular disease risk.
— Bake, broil, steam or grill foods. Avoid frying to reduce calories and fat.
• Exercise as able. Consider adaptive exercise equipment, such as arm ergometry (similar to pedaling a bicycle with the arms), FES leg biking or swimming.
• Avoid smoking and secondhand smoke.
• Reduce stress.

Lungs and Respiratory System

Aging lungs lose the ability to exchange as much oxygen and carbon dioxide as they once did. The reason is a natural reduction in the air sacs (alveoli) in the lungs. The lungs also become less elastic, and the muscles used in filling the chest cavity with air become weaker and stiffer. Loss of breathing capacity results in additional difficulty fighting off infections, such as pneumonia, influenza (flu) and even the common cold.

Respiratory problems are more common in people with SCI, especially those with high-level injuries who have reduced lung capacity. Many people with SCI may have trouble coughing or clearing their lungs, which typically worsens with age. Those with tetraplegia who rely on a ventilator to help them breathe have a greater risk of developing infections.

To help prevent lung or respiratory system problems:
• Perform deep breathing exercises twice daily; increase frequency if you have a cold
• Maintain adequate hydration
• Get influenza vaccinations annually and pneumonia vaccines as directed by your provider
• Avoid smoke and pollution
• Maintain a healthy body weight

Sleep apnea

The risk of sleep apnea (pauses in breathing while sleeping) increases with tetraplegia, age and obesity. You may also have shortness of breath if you are overweight, have spine deformities (scoliosis or kyphosis), or chest wall or abdominal spasticity. See *Respiratory Care*, Chapter Two, for additional information.

Gastrointestinal System

Most changes that occur in the gastrointestinal (GI) or digestive system are so subtle that they may not be noticeable. Swallowing and the motions that automatically move digested food through the intestines slow with age. The flow of secretions from the stomach, liver, pancreas and small intestine also may decrease.

For those with SCI, food takes longer to pass through the GI tract. Constipation (passage of hard stools less than three times per week) and more time for bowel care can result. Constipation can also be caused by poor diet, dehydration, medications, inactivity or illness. Passing hard stools may be difficult and painful. Hemorrhoids (swelling of the veins in the anus) or a bowel obstruction sometimes result. Hemorrhoids can occur after long periods of sitting or digital stimulation during your bowel management program. The major sign of hemorrhoids is bleeding during your bowel management program.

Other common GI problems include stool impaction, distention (swelling) of the colon, abdominal bloating, prolonged or incomplete emptying of the bowel, an unproductive bowel program, incontinence or gallstones.

To help prevent GI problems:
- Maintain adequate hydration and a high fiber diet
- Review your bowel program with your health care provider and modify as necessary. You may need to increase the frequency of your program to daily or every other day as recommended
- Maintain as active a lifestyle as possible
- Request a colorectal cancer screening at age 50

Urinary System

Aging may be accompanied by more frequent urination or catheterization. Holding your urine or emptying your bladder may become more difficult. Inability to hold your urine can result in leakage or incontinence. A bladder that is not completely empty can lead to infections. Aging with SCI places you at higher risk of urinary tract infections, bladder and kidney stones, kidney infection, kidney failure and bladder cancer.

Kidney function declines with age and must be watched closely after SCI. At about age 40, you begin to lose some of the important filters, called nephrons, within the kidneys. This gradual decline in kidney function can be a problem for those who take medications or have a chronic illness, such as high blood pressure or diabetes. A severe decline or stop in function, called kidney failure, is becoming more common because people are living longer with chronic illnesses that can harm their kidneys. The damage done by kidney failure is irreversible and requires dialysis (removal of waste products from the blood and excess fluid from the body). Therefore, it is extremely important to follow up with your health care provider on a yearly basis when you have SCI.

To help prevent urinary system problems:
- Keep anal and genital areas clean and dry
- Get prompt treatment for bladder infections
- Have yearly urologic evaluations to assess kidney and bladder function
- Adhere to your prescribed bladder management program
- Review your bladder management program with your health care provider and modify as necessary
- Follow your prescribed fluid program closely, assuring adequate fluid intake
- Discuss any new medication with your care provider to rule out any adverse effects on the kidneys

Nervous System

Aging contributes to loss or decline of some sensations, muscle mass and strength. The result can be slower reaction time, decreased fine motor coordination and less stability while walking. These changes may increase the difficulty of performing everyday activities and the risk of falls. The nervous system also controls your internal body temperature. As you age, malfunctioning body temperature controls can make you feel hotter or colder even in normal room temperatures.

Some persons may develop pain syndromes, such as muscle or joint pain. Nerve pain, also known as neuropathic or central pain, can occur after SCI, especially in persons with incomplete injuries. This pain is typically characterized as tightness, pressure, burning, cold, heaviness, numbness, or a pins-and-needles feeling. These sensations can be continuous and may fluctuate in intensity. Several medication treatment options are available, such as tricyclic antidepressants (amitriptyline, nortriptyline), anticonvulsants (gabapentin, pregabalin), nonsteroidal anti-inflammatory drugs, capsaicin cream, or opioids. Non-medicinal interventions may include spinal cord stimulation, acupuncture and transcutaneous electrical stimulation (TENS), a portable device that provides electrical impulses to nerves through the skin. Talk to your health care provider to determine if medicinal or non-medicinal treatment is an option.

As you age with SCI, you may notice a decline in function, strength and sensation. One cause may be syringomyelia, the progressive enlargement of a spinal cord cyst, which can develop near your injury site. This condition is confirmed by magnetic resonance imaging (MRI) and may require surgery.

Signs and symptoms of syringomyelia include:
- Loss of motor and sensory function
- Increased spasticity
- Neuropathic pain
- Sweating
- Increased episodes of autonomic hyperreflexia

Overuse can also lead to nerve compression, such as carpal tunnel syndrome or hand numbness from pressure on the ulnar nerve around the elbow. In addition, herniation (abnormal protrusion of tissue through an opening) in the back or neck may lead to new pains or weakness. Periodic sensory or motor-skill evaluations by your health care provider are important.

To help prevent nervous system problems:
- Discuss pain management with your health care provider.
- Modify or obtain adaptive equipment.
- Watch for changes in strength, sensation or function. Notify your health care provider if changes occur.

Functional Changes

Besides the physical affects that aging can have on your body, there are other considerations that you must be aware of. Aging can affect your independence. As the SCI population ages, typically their caregivers are also aging. Therefore, as performing the tasks of daily living become more difficult, caregivers can find that doing these tasks for you is more difficult. You may need to look at different ways to achieve tasks, acquire new equipment (such as a power wheelchair or lift), and obtain new or additional care attendants. Finances may also be more of a burden due to the cost of additional hospitalizations, prescription drugs, supplies and institutional care. Your social worker can help.

Because of the physical and functional changes that can occur with aging, especially after SCI, it is important to attend annual spinal cord-specific evaluations. These evaluations also screen for secondary complications of aging. Report any problems to your health care provider to avoid secondary complications. If you are hospitalized, talk to the treating health care provider about your special SCI-related needs to ensure appropriate care.

Anticipate the changes caused by aging. Practice healthy living behaviors, acquire new skills, use new equipment, incorporate the assistance of others, alter your priorities and change attitudes. Doing so can allow you to live a long healthy life after spinal cord injury.

Living Fully with a
Spinal Cord Injury

8 Actively Participating in Your Life

GOING BACK TO WORK

Work is defined as productive activity. Work plays a major role in the lives of most individuals and provides many benefits, such as achievement, responsibility, recognition, variety, financial independence, social status, and structure. Those who continue to work after spinal cord injury are generally healthier, have higher self-esteem and spend less time in the hospital than those who do not work. Work allows you to express your personality.

Returning to paid employment is an important concern for those with SCI. Regardless of whether or not you return to work, your main task after SCI is to discover how to use your talents in spite of your injury. Expressing your talents may be done through paid employment, volunteer, or other nonvocational activities. What you do will depend on your situation.

People with SCI work in many occupations. The type of job you can perform will depend on your physical capabilities. Your physical limitations may prevent you from returning to your former job, or require that you shift from working with things (physical objects) to working with data (words and/or numbers), or people. For instance, people with tetraplegia (quadriplegia) often work with data, since this type of position is usually less physically demanding. People with paraplegia, however, may find they work more easily with physical objects.

All jobs require dealing with either data, people, things, or a combination of all three. Think about the jobs you have had and which you enjoyed the most.

This chapter can assist you in making decisions about re-entering the work force by:

- Describing how to assess your personal interest and aptitudes when returning to work
- Providing ideas on finding a job and describing resources that are available to help you
- Identifying planning concepts to review before returning to the work setting

Factors to Consider

Returning to work after SCI depends on factors such as:

- Availability of jobs
- Your health
- Your physical abilities
- Your motivation
- Vocational interests and aptitudes
- Willingness to complete further training
- Willingness of employers to adapt the job or workplace
- Impact on disability pension benefits
- Impact on health insurance coverage

By understanding the structure of the work world and your skills as a worker, you can better match yourself to the right job.

Interests

If you cannot return to the job you had before your spinal cord injury, you may want to evaluate your interests in order to decide what kind of job you can and want to do. List the activities, jobs and school subjects that you enjoyed before your injury. These interests may provide ideas for work.

Interests can also be evaluated through psychological tests, called interest inventories. Interest inventories list many jobs, school subjects, types of people and activities. Your response to these items is compared to the response of people happily employed in specific jobs. The more similar your interests are to those already employed, the greater the chance that you would like doing that work.

Aptitudes

Aptitudes are natural abilities to perform certain mental or physical tasks with ease. They can be divided into three broad categories:

- *Cognitive:* Problem solving using words and numbers
- *Perceptual:* Problem solving using vision

- *Psychomotor:* Physical speed and skill

One way to determine your current aptitudes is to take an aptitude test. Rehabilitation psychologists or vocational counselors are trained to provide this service and may already be part of your rehabilitation team. Your results can be matched to those of people employed in many job areas. Your matches can help you select a job category that offers you the most likelihood for success.

The Job Market

Due to global competition, new technology and changes in the work force, Americans are now more likely to change jobs several times during their careers. Job-search skills have become very important. However, the more training you complete, the easier it is to find work. Therefore, it is important to further your education if possible.

How to Find a Job

Success in finding a job requires effective job-search strategies. You must determine job openings and how to get an interview. Some options include:

- Gathering detailed and reliable information from published and human sources about jobs. You might search for publications that provide current information on job descriptions, training needed to do specific jobs and the predicted demand for jobs in the future. You can also talk to a person who performs a certain job, for information about that job. The Occupational Information Network (O*NET available at www.online.onetcenter. org) provides a comprehensive database of worker attributes and job characteristics. The federal government's Bureau of Labor Statistics web site has links to current information on the U.S. economy. The Occupational Outlook Handbook describes the job duties, working conditions, training and educational requirements, earnings, and job prospects for 260 of the most common occupations in the U.S. See the *Additional Information* section at the end of the book, for more information.
- Maintaining contacts with friends and family, since they can be primary sources of finding employment. Tell them that you are looking for work, and explain the type of work that is compatible with your SCI.
- Increasing your social contacts by joining civic, religious, and business groups where you might meet potential employers.

Employers prefer to know as much as possible about an applicant before the interview. In addition, these activities are viewed favorably on a job application.

- Contacting local employers and asking them to keep your job application or resume on file in case they have a job opening. If you are working with a state vocational rehabilitation agency, the agency may be able to provide sources of employment. Other possible sources include private employment agencies and listings in professional and trade publications.
- Checking jobs listed in newspapers or with your state's employment service.

Effective Job Interviews

You can increase your chances of being hired for a job by:
- Learning as much as possible about the job requirements
- Submitting a well-written resume
- Providing good references

Remember these tips for a successful interview:
- Your appearance should be neat and well-groomed.
- Put the interviewer at ease.
- Be confident.
- Emphasize your abilities.
- Be positive about your needs and limitations.
- Know how you will get to and from work.
- Subtly emphasize that you do not want a favor, you want an equal chance.
- Emphasize your awareness of job responsibilities such as being on time, working well with others, and avoiding excessive absences.
- Know your rights offered by legislation such as the Americans with Disabilities Act (see The American with Disabilities Act of 1990, at the end of this chapter, for more information), but do not threaten the interviewer with this knowledge.

Some state and private employment agencies supply tip sheets on resume writing and preparing for interviews.

Can I Afford to Work?

One of the most perplexing questions you will face is whether you can afford to work. In most cases, after SCI you are provided an income that covers your basic necessities. This income, together with housing, health and sometimes attendant care benefits, complicates the return-to-work decision. You may face losing health care or other benefits if you earn more than a certain income. A potential job must pay enough (at least a low to moderate income) and have adequate health insurance coverage to make having the job financially realistic.

Know the rules regarding state and federal programs that cover you. For more information, see the resources section at the end of the book. Learn how much you can earn before benefits are reduced or stopped. Determine if there is a trial work period during which you can receive benefits. This will help you decide if the job is appropriate. Talk to your current or potential employer for additional information.

Sources of Vocational Help

Vocational rehabilitation

Each state has a Division of Vocational Rehabilitation responsible for helping people with disabilities achieve their vocational goals. Employment can be in the competitive labor market, in a self-owned business, at home, or in some cases in the role of a homemaker. Services may include physical and vocational evaluations, assistive devices, training, transportation and placement assistance.

The typical process begins with you contacting your state's vocational rehabilitation service and by telephone, setting up an appointment to meet with an intake worker, which includes filling out an application for services. Once documentation of your disability is submitted and you are formally approved for services, a state vocational rehabilitation counselor will contact you for an appointment and devise a return to work plan. You will meet with the counselor as needed. Talk to your state's Department of Vocational Rehabilitation for more information.

Other sources

If you are a veteran, the Veterans Administration (VA) has a Vocational Rehabilitation Program which provides services similar to those offered by a state agency. Career counseling services also are offered through local vocational-technical institutes, community colleges, or four-year colleges and universities. Frequently, these schools have counseling staff that specialize in helping those with disabilities.

Planning Your Return to Work

Returning to work is very rewarding, but may take some advance planning. You may want to:

- Determine if you can return to your previous work position.
- If so, discuss with your Human Resources department ways it can assist in your return.
- Start with reduced work hours.
- Evaluate the accessibility of the work space.
  - Parking
  - Access into the building
  - Desk and meeting room table clearance for your wheelchair
  - Turning radius for wheelchair in work setting, meeting rooms, bathrooms, breakrooms, lounges, and cafeterias
  - Access to co-workers
  - Accessible restrooms
- Inquire about adaptive equipment.
  - Computer accessories, voice controls
  - Phone accessories
- Plan for personal care.
  - Find clean, large, well-lit area to perform self-catheterization if needed
  - Package and bring supplies needed during the work shift
  - Assure time is allowed for you to perform personal care
  - Plan for accidents or incidents
- Plan that you may be the only person around at times.
  - Assure light switches, fax machines and photocopiers are within your reach
  - Assure that you can open the necessary doors

LEISURE/RECREATION

Recreation and leisure time is an important part of your life and can be rewarding following spinal cord injury. After SCI, you may think that you can no longer participate in activities you enjoyed previously. However, with adaptations and special equipment, you may resume many activities, including sports.

Importance of Leisure/Recreational Activities

Physical activity can be fun and help maintain total body health. Leisure activities also can help you meet people and strengthen friendships. Hobbies can improve your self-esteem and increase your self-confidence. Participating in fun activities can decrease stress and help you relax.

Available Activities

You can still do many activities you enjoyed before your disability. You may also choose to try some new ones. The activities you pursue will depend on:

- Your interests
- Your physical abilities
- Activities that are available in your community
- Your creativity
- Your motivation to try new things

Be creative and find new ways to do things. Your disability should not hinder you.

Getting Back into the Community

Your disability may cause you to feel uneasy about going out in public, which is natural. People might treat you differently than before your disability, which is also common. They may stare, ignore you, or talk to you as if you are less intelligent. Their reactions may not be what they seem. These reactions can be caused by feelings of uncertainty, not an intention to be unkind. You may need to assert yourself and take control of social situations. Try to put others at ease. How you act influences how others react. Social interactions will become easier over time, as you become more comfortable with your condition.

Back at home, it is important to seek out and maintain involvement with others in the community. Your activities will require more planning, so use resources for people with disabilities, such as your city's recreational department or YMCA. In smaller communities, finding opportunities for leisure/recreation may require more creativity.

Sources of activities may include:

- Schools
- Community education
- Sports arenas
- Malls
- Civic centers
- Hospitals

- Service organizations
- Bowling leagues
- Sports clubs
- Parks
- Theaters
- Restaurants
- United Way organizations
- Clubs
- Libraries
- Centers for Independent Living
- Boy/Girl Scout organizations

Call ahead to see if facilities are wheelchair-accessible.

Wheelchair Sports

Many people who have disabilities enjoy recreational and competitive wheelchair sports. These sports can help you maintain physical health and mental well-being through exercise, which increases blood flow and maintains your strength. Hand-eye coordination and breathing also improve through exercise. Good conditioning helps your body resist minor illness, and often helps you handle the wheelchair more skillfully.

The popularity and participants in wheelchair sports continue to increase, as does the number of sports available. Some sports done either in or out of a wheelchair include:
- Archery
- Basketball
- Biking
- Bowling
- Canoeing
- Golf
- Horseback riding
- Road racing/marathons
- Rock climbing
- Rugby
- Skiing
- Softball
- Swimming
- Tennis
- Track and field

The competition and teamwork that various wheelchair sports offer can help you reach your fullest potential. The satisfaction that comes from these sports, both recreational and competitive, can increase your feelings of self-worth and self-esteem.

Many communities have competitions in organized wheelchair sports. To be fair, competition in wheelchair sports is divided into medical disability classes. Whether you compete or enjoy the activity privately, wheelchair sports are sources of great enjoyment and self-satisfaction.

It Is Up to You

The decision to find and become involved in leisure/recreational opportunities is yours. If you do not seek out opportunities in your community, you may never realize the good experiences you missed. Tell others about your leisure/recreational needs and interests. Find ways to maximize your abilities while doing what you enjoy.

TRAVEL INFORMATION

If you are physically disabled, traveling can be a special challenge. By planning your trip carefully, you can increase your confidence and travel enjoyment. The purpose of this material is to provide you with information about different methods of travel, including suggestions for planning a trip by land, air or sea, as well as lodging recommendations.

General Information

Below are some general suggestions to follow when planning a trip:
- Plan well in advance to avoid mix-ups and confusion. You might want to make a daily log of what to do and items you may need.
- Search the Internet for information about accessibility for the disabled at your destination.
- Call for accessible hotel or motel and transportation reservations well ahead of your travel date.
- When planning a trip by air or train, you may want to ask a local travel agent to assist with your reservations. Make your needs very clear to the travel agent.
- Ask for transportation between the terminal entrance and departure gates if you need it. Depending on your special needs, some plane or train seating may not be possible. Ask the reservation person to book a seat that is accessible to you.

- Always allow enough time for travel. Arrive at the plane or train terminal at least two hours before departure. Book long layovers, since wheelchair users are typically first on and last off of planes or trains.
- Always reconfirm your airline reservations at least one day before leaving. If you use E-tickets, you can check your reservations online.
- When traveling by vehicle, remember that driving in the winter can be hazardous and you should be prepared for bad weather. Carry a cell phone, warm clothing, blankets and an emergency kit in your vehicle. This kit should include flares, candles, matches, a shovel, self-care supplies (catheter kit, etc.), first aid kit, blankets, water and storable food.

Travel By Land

Private transportation

Car

Select a car that meets your needs. Be sure that you can get into and out of the car easily. You may need hand controls to drive. Driver's training can be arranged through your social worker or local Center for Independent Living.

Vans

Vans are a good option if you have a power wheelchair or have problems transferring from your wheelchair. They can be equipped with one of several types of electric or hydraulic lifts. The lift can be placed either on the side or in back of the van (the side mount is most popular).

Parking

There are designated parking areas for people with disabilities. To park in these places, you must either have a handicapped license plate or a special parking certificate placed on your visor. Check with your state's Department of Vehicle Registration for more information about parking specifics.

Public (local transportation)

Cab or private van companies

Cabs in many cities provide wheelchair services. You can transfer from your wheelchair to the cab, or you can remain in your wheelchair if using a wheelchair cab. A wheelchair cab usually does not cost extra. Some private van companies specialize in transportation for persons with disabilities. You may consider this option if you have a hard time transferring from your wheelchair. Check under transportation services in the phonebook or Internet for additional information.

Bus

Public buses accommodate people with disabilities who have mobility problems. Federal law states that people with disabilities must have equal access to public transportation. However, local governments have the authority to decide if transportation for those with disabilities are a fixed route or a Dial-a-Ride system. Check with your local bus company for more information.

Dial-a-Ride

Some cities offer subsidized transportation services for people with disabilities. You must apply and qualify for the service. In some cities, to schedule a ride, you must notify the Dial-a-Ride Service at least 24 hours in advance. If offered, Dial-a-Ride information can be found under transportation or bus services in the phonebook or Internet.

Rental car or van services

Rental car or van services differ among companies. In general, you will need to call at least five days in advance to reserve a vehicle with hand controls. There may be an extra charge. Make sure you specify left-hand or right-hand controls. Global positioning systems (GPS) are helpful for navigation, but may cost extra. Some companies require that you return the vehicle to the place where you picked it up.

When renting a car, you usually will need a major credit card. For cash rentals, you typically need to make a deposit. This deposit is returned to you or credited toward your final bill when you return the vehicle. Ask about other rental details when you call for reservations.

Public (city-to-city transportation)

Bus

Some bus services allow you to bring along an attendant or travel companion whose fare is either free or a reduced cost. To qualify, you may need a written statement from your doctor that a companion is needed for physical assistance in bus travel. You should call 48 hours in advance to request boarding assistance. Some bus companies have wheelchair-lift buses; others may have alternative lift equipment. Aisles are narrow and restrooms are usually small and located at the back of the bus.

Accessible terminals vary from city to city. Verify that the terminals along your trip route have the services you need. You may need to change terminals, so plan a route with the fewest changes.

Travel By Train

When you travel by train, a conductor may help you get on and off. Trains have a varying degree of accessibility. Some trains have wheelchair-accessible cars, dining areas and sleep areas. For seating, it is sometimes recommended that you transfer from your wheelchair to a regular seat. Aisles are typically narrow, and going from one car to another can be hard. Walking on a moving train can be difficult, so you may request to have your meal brought to your seat or compartment. If you bring an attendant or companion, inquire about discount fares for companions. Ask a travel agent or the train company what accommodations are available.

Travel By Air

Reservations information

To avoid complications, make your reservations as far in advance of your travel date as possible. When making reservations yourself or through a travel agent, ask for seats closest to the front of the aircraft, in either first class or economy. Airlines are required to give disabled persons first chance at bulkhead seats (the first seats in coach). The transfer to and from your wheelchair is easier with these seats. Request to be upgraded to first class when you arrive at the departure gate. Often, the upgrade is free if there is an open seat. The following diagram can help you locate ideal seating in first class or economy (Figure 1).

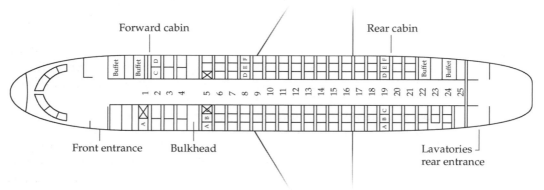

Figure 1. Ideal seating on an airplane (indicated by an "X").

Airpc

Airport ac
the airport b

Getting on and

Concourse approache
the aircraft with little d
can travel down a series of
try. If there is a large step to th
have the concourse adjusted. So
aisle chair (a narrow chair that fits   ard
the plane even if there is an accessible

With step-way aircraft entry, a movable   flush with
the aircraft. You must transfer from your wh   to a narrower
aisle chair. This chair is carried up the step-way   to the plane cabin
by airline personnel and then is moved to the assigned seat.

Manual wheelchair storage

Your wheelchair can be checked at the ticket counter or gate. You
can request to have your wheelchair stowed on board when pre-
boarding. Your wheelchair will be stored in the plane's baggage
compartment. Some wheelchair suppliers keep packing boxes and
may have one available for transporting your chair.

Before storage, make sure all arms and legs are locked firmly in
place. Remove wheelchair cushions and backpacks and carry them
on board. With a tag, those unloading the baggage will know that
you want the wheelchair as soon as possible. It will also inform them
to bring it to the concourse you are getting off on. Before landing at
your destination, have the cabin attendant call ahead to the ground
crew and request that they take your wheelchair to the concourse immediately after arrival. That allows you to deplane without delay.

Crutches, canes and other walking aids that may be carried on board
are placed in a special compartment for safety reasons. Should you
need these during the flight, ask your cabin attendant to get them.

Power wheelchair storage

Power wheelchairs are generally not disassembled for transportation, unless they do not fit upright through the aircraft cargo
door. Batteries on power wheelchairs must be identified as 'spillable' or 'non-spillable' due to federal regulations. Spillable (wet-cell)

…ected and terminals protected against elec-
…e battery may need to be shipped in the aircraft
…to meet federal regulations.

Non-spillable (dry-cell or gel-cell) batteries can remain attached to the power wheelchair when the equipment fits upright through the aircraft cargo department door. Airline personnel may disconnect the battery post connectors and wrap each post with tape to prevent electrical shorts during transportation. Ask your airline if it will transport your battery along with your chair. You may need to arrange for a battery to be waiting at your destination.

Changing planes en route

Sometimes, when you travel long distances, you may have to change flights en route to your final destination. If possible, try to stay on the same airline for your entire trip. This can help eliminate long trips to other airline concourses at major airports. If required, request transportation between gates.

Determine if you have layovers on your flight. A travel agent who handles your reservations should inform you about layovers. Know the length of the layover, the name of the transfer airline and how long it takes to get to the terminal of departure. If the layover is for an extended time (2 to 3 hours), some air terminals may have a rest area where you may relax between flights. Find out this information before your trip to make travel easier.

Notify the airline in advance if you prefer to use your own personal wheelchair at the connecting airport. Due to time constraints and disassemble/reassemble of your wheelchair, this service may not be feasible during your layover. You may want to take advantage of airline's service instead.

Restrooms on planes

Restrooms on most planes are not very accessible for people with disabilities. Many are too small either for an aisle chair to fit into, or to transfer into. One alternative option may be to wear a urine collection device. Talk to a member of your health care team for information about alternative options. Be sure to urinate (void) before boarding the plane.

Baggage

If you are unable to handle your baggage by yourself, ask representatives to arrange for airport personnel help you.

Travel By Sea

During the last 10 years, many on-board improvements have made ships more accessible to people with disabilities. Choose passenger ships with accessible staterooms, ramps and elevators. Request a cabin near the elevator. Ask for help from the ship's crew when boarding and leaving.

For more specific information on accessibility, costs and departure dates, search the Internet or consult a travel agent.

Lodging

Many chain motels or hotels have toll-free numbers for reserving a wheelchair-accessible room in advance. Ask about accessibility. For example, a roll-in shower is not a standard feature in accessible rooms. Make your reservations as far in advance of your travel date as possible to guarantee an accessible room and bathroom. When making reservations, ask if the pool, recreation room, party room, restaurants and public bathrooms are also accessible.

MAINTAINING YOUR EQUIPMENT

Proper care for the equipment you use following spinal cord injury is very important. Maintenance requirements vary greatly depending on the item and the manufacturer. Proper care helps ensures that your equipment is safe, works as intended, and lasts longer.

Wheelchair Cushions

Cushions increase your comfort and help relieve pressure on your skin. Many types of cushions are available. Ask your therapist to recommend a cushion that will best meet your needs. Below are guidelines for proper care and use of different cushions.

Air-filled (Roho™)
The air cells of this cushion surround and support your sitting area so your body weight is distributed evenly over the cushion's surface.

Advantages:
- Lightweight
- Easy to clean
- Maximum pressure distribution

- Reduces shear (skin damage that occurs when your skin moves in one direction and the bone underneath moves in another)

Disadvantages:
- Poor sitting stability
- Subject to puncture
- Difficult to repair

Tips:
- Check the cushion daily for leaks and decreases in pressure, especially with changes in altitude or extreme temperature changes.
- Learn to inflate your cushion properly so it will effectively relieve pressure on your skin. Talk to your therapist about how to properly inflate your cushion.

Foam
A variety of foam cushions are available in either a flat or contoured design. Talk to your therapist about which design is best.

Advantages:
- Relatively inexpensive
- Easy to use
- Easy to modify
- Contour cushions help position the body properly

Disadvantages:
- Wears out faster
- Hard to clean
- Traps body heat

Tips:
- You may need to replace the foam every 9 to 12 months if it becomes compressed or deteriorates—the sitting area hardens, loses thickness and doesn't spring back when your weight is removed.
- Using a cushion cover may help prevent your cushion from becoming moist and smelling badly.
- If your cushion has a cutout, be certain that the cushion is placed properly in the wheelchair and that you sit on it correctly.

Flat gel (Action Pad ™)
A flat gel cushion conforms to body contours and can reduce shearing in active people.

Advantages:
- Reduces shear
- Provides shock absorption
- Easy to clean

Disadvantages:
- Heavy
- Traps body heat
- Provides little pressure relief for those who have decreased sensation

Tips:
- Rotate the cushion one-fourth turn every day if the cushion is square. If it is rectangular, rotate the cushion one-half turn every day.
- You may need to replace the cushion if it becomes compressed, firm or thick around the edges.

Jay Cushion™
Gel and foam combination cushion.

Advantages:
- Stable positioning
- Reduces shear
- Shock absorption
- Easy to clean

Disadvantages:
- Heavy
- Gel may migrate away from bony areas
- Can be placed incorrectly
- Traps body heat
- Freezes in subfreezing temperatures

Tips:
- Check the fluid for proper consistency
- Check the pad for punctures

Wheelchairs

Each wheelchair requires different maintenance. Check your owner's manual for specific recommendations and warranty information. If you have questions, contact your therapist or wheelchair vendor. Below are general guidelines for wheelchair care.

Manual wheelchair

Weekly
- Check the tire pressure with a gauge and keep the tires inflated to the recommended pressure.
- Check the valve system. If air leaks out around the valve, tighten the stem with a forked metal cap (available at bike shops).

Monthly
- Use all-purpose oil to lubricate the crossbrace.
- Clean the upholstery; check for tears, cracks and overstretching.

Six months
- Check the wheel alignment or have the wheelchair serviced by a vendor.
- Check tire wear and replace tires if necessary.
- Tighten the wheel lugs and screws on the upholstery and handrims.

Yearly
- Have your wheelchair serviced and cleaned by a wheelchair vendor. The vendor may loan you a wheelchair while servicing yours.
- Check for any loose bolts or screws.

Power wheelchair
- Follow your owner's manual for regularly scheduled maintenance.
- Maintain battery charge daily.
- Install and maintain batteries according to instructions in the owner's manual.
- Check monthly for loose bolts or screws.
- Contact your wheelchair vendor if you hear unusual noises coming from the wheelchair.

Lower Extremity Orthotics (Braces)

With braces, standing and walking may be possible and may help you access rooms, buildings and high places that may be otherwise inaccessible. In addition to providing mobility, braces can help increase cardiovascular fitness and decrease the possibility of developing osteoporosis. Osteoporosis is a condition caused by the loss of calcium and other substances from bones, causing bones to become thin, brittle and more likely to fracture. Weight-bearing exercise and activity helps strengthen bones.

Braces can be dependable and fairly trouble-free. However, some daily care is required. Use the following guidelines to help keep your braces in good working condition and to make those minor adjustments that do not require a specialist.

Daily checklist

- Check your skin for irritation, especially at points of contact between your skin and the brace.
- Check buckles, straps, laces and Velcro™ for wear.
- Tighten loose screws or rivets or contact your brace specialist to replace missing ones.
- Check the joints and locks for smooth, safe operation.
- Check your shoes for excessive wear on the soles or heels. Excessive wear may affect your balance and the adjustment of the brace.

Metal parts of the brace

- Wipe aluminum parts occasionally with a soft cloth.
- Check for nicks or rough spots.
- Check for loose or missing screws or nuts.

Plastic parts, plastic splints and braces

- Plastic should be cleaned regularly with a cloth dipped in rubbing alcohol.
- Be sure there are no rough areas where the plastic touches your skin.

Upper Extremity Orthotics (Splints)

Upper extremity orthotics, or splints, can prevent unwanted changes in the hands and arms, and may increase a person's functional ability. Splints fabricated by occupational therapists in the hospital are usually made with low temperature thermoplastics that typically last for months and sometimes years. These include resting hand splints and wrist supports. Orthotists will often provide commercial or fabricate splints of more durable materials, which can last for years. These include an adjustable elbow extension or a wrist driven tenodesis splint.

All splints require routine care and careful observation for signs of wear and improper fit. Bring your splints to spinal cord injury health care provider follow-up appointments.

Wearing schedule

Follow the splint-wearing schedule as instructed by your therapist and/or health care provider. If you notice reddened areas on your skin or feel discomfort, contact your therapist.

Avoid damage

Keep your splint away from direct heat, such as car heaters, stoves, radiators or intense sunlight. Otherwise, your splint may soften and lose its shape. Since pets often like to chew on splints, keep your splint away from them.

Routine wear

Your splint should be cleaned daily, wiping it with a clean, warm washcloth. Soiling can be removed by gently washing with a liquid soap and rinsing with cool water. Over time Velcro straps and attachments may need to be cleaned or replaced. Splint materials can also age, becoming discolored, deformed or cracked. If this should occur, you should contact your therapist to have your splint checked, repaired or replaced.

Precautions

Do not adjust or modify your own splint with padding, cushions or other materials.

Assistive Technology Devices

Following a spinal cord injury, people will often experience a loss of function that affects their ability to perform important tasks and fulfill a variety of roles and responsibilities. Regaining control and independence is a critical part of rehabilitation. The first priority of rehabilitation is to reduce the impact of the injury, such as restoring strength, range of motion, endurance. Unfortunately, there are almost always lasting physical problems that can affect a person's arms, legs or both. These problems can interfere with the ability to care for yourself, take care of work in the home and community, or engage in meaningful leisure activities.

Assistive devices are tools that allow someone with functional limitations to perform jobs or tasks more independently. Without these tools, a person with SCI may need to depend on a caregiver or personal care assistant to perform self-care, work or leisure activities. As physical skills are regained, there may no longer be a need for assistive devices, or less assistance may be needed. For example, as leg strength improves, there may be progression from using a wheelchair to a walker or cane.

Aids to daily living

One of the first areas addressed after SCI are self-care skills. These include eating, grooming, dressing, bathing and toileting. There are a wide range of assistive devices that can help someone regain their independence with these tasks. The assistive devices used depend on what tasks the person needs to do and his or her abilities. An occupational therapist can help you improve your abilities and teach you to use assistive devices to bridge the gap between what you can do and what you need to do. This process begins in the hospital and progresses through rehabilitation, to the home and community. Assistive devices compensate and help restore the loss of strength, active range of motion and endurance, as well as restoring independence.

- *Eating:* Adaptive eating utensils and devices can be used when the upper body is affected by SCI (tetraplegia). These utensils support the arms, such as a mobile arm support or deltoid aid. A non-skid pad can hold a plate or bowl in place. To prevent food from sliding off the plate or utensil, a plate guard or inner lip plate can be used.

- *Grooming:* Placing a toothbrush in a utensil cuff, using a flip-top toothpaste tube or an adapted dental floss holder can assist with oral hygiene care. Long-handled combs or brushes with Velcro straps can be used for hair care. Electric and blade razors can be adapted if there is some control of the upper arms, but limited hand function.

- *Bathing:* Having a safe sitting surface for bathing is important regardless of the level of injury. Shower chairs are an assistive device that works well if you can stand and transfer, since using a shower chair requires stepping over a tub or shower threshold. If you have fairly good trunk control and transfer abilities, a tub or shower transfer bench works well. If there is a loss of sensation or a concern about the skin, then a padded seat and back may be very important. A high level spinal cord injury will likely require a shower chair commode, sometimes with chest supports and a recline feature. These require a roll-in shower and additional room for you and a caregiver. If some hand control is present, but there is difficulty reaching, a long-handled sponge wash mitt or hand-held shower may be all that is needed for independent bathing.

- *Dressing:* Completion of upper body dressing without adaptive equipment if possible for a person when the lower body is affected by SCI (paraplegia). However, dressing your lower body may be more difficult, particularly with decreased hip and back range of motion. In these situations a reacher, dressing stick, sock aid, or slip-on shoes may be all that is required. For people with SCI that affects control of the upper body and trunk, there may be much greater challenges, perhaps requiring the aid of a caregiver or dressing in bed. Nevertheless, there are several tasks that may be possible with the right training and equipment. For example, pull-over shirts, Velcro fasteners, a button hook or zipper puller and loops on pants may ease some dressing tasks.

- *Toileting:* The ability to independently manage bowel and bladder care is often a high priority after SCI. If you can transfer onto a regular toilet, a riser, grab bars or toilet safety frame, and widened doorways are often sufficient. If it is difficult reaching to wipe, a toilet aid often works. A suppository inserter or digital stimulator to assist with initiating a bowel movement may be used. If you use a leg bag but cannot empty it yourself, an electric leg bag valve may allow you empty the bag in public without others knowing.

Home and environmental modifications

One of the first questions asked when someone is admitted to a rehabilitation unit is, "Where are you going to go after you leave the hospital?" The hospital has even floors in hallways, wide doors, accessible bathrooms and meals delivered to your room. For most people with a spinal cord injury, home is not always that convenient. While not all homes can be made wheelchair accessible, there are a number of modifications that may make it possible and convenient for you to return to your home. It is important to discuss your home's accessibility with your therapists before you begin any major remodeling projects. They may be able to save you time and money, as well as making your home work for you.

- *Stairs, ramps and lifts:* Independently entering and leaving the home can not only be frustrating, it can also be a safety hazard in an emergency. For someone using a walker, wide, shallow steps or a ramp with a gentle slope can be a practical home modification. For homes with little room for a ramp, a wheelchair lift (similar to a short elevator) may be the only option. There are also residential elevators and stair lifts available to meet a wide range of home design challenges when it is necessary to access more than a single level of a home. In some communities, the local Center for Independent Living may be able to help with the design, construction and cost of ramps and lifts.

- *Bathroom modifications:* Because of the confined space of most bathrooms, many people with a SCI will consider a bathroom makeover. Before beginning, talking to your occupational therapist and discussing the space and functional limitations of your bathroom may be beneficial. A combination of grab bars, toilet risers, wheel-in showers, curtains instead of doors, transfer tub benches and other modifications may be suggested. However, improvement in transfer ability or simple modifications may help avoid the need for a major remodeling.

- *Transfer equipment:* Safe transfers involve getting from one point to another safely and efficiently, while also protecting your arms, back and skin. When considering safe transfers, the safety of your caregivers is also important. Training in the use and the proper selection of sliding boards or patient lifts is best accomplished by your physical or occupational therapist. Any equipment used for transfers must be safe and durable. You should check your equipment every time you transfer and keep up on regular maintenance.

- *Kitchen and home adaptations:* Meal preparation and using the kitchen is an important daily home management activity. Whether someone uses a wheelchair or walker, reaching into deep shelves or cupboards and carrying items can be difficult and potentially unsafe. Open cabinets, pullout shelving, turntables and bins, and a variety of storage options are readily available at home improvement stores. Removing the doors from cupboards under the sink may provide wheelchair access. Roll-under cook tops, oven sticks, above stove mirrors, adapted cutting boards and cooking utensils can make cooking and meal preparation easier and safer. Using a walker, walker basket/tray or rolling cart can make it easier and safer to carry items between the refrigerator, meal preparation and dining areas.

- Other environmental adaptations to consider in your home:
  - Look at obstacles that could be a tripping hazard or make propelling a wheelchair more difficult.
  - Remove throw rugs.
  - Install low height thresholds or remove thresholds.
  - Install angled door hinges which can increase door width by 1 to 2 inches.
  - Apply trim along walls and at corners which can protect the walls from wheelchair strikes.
  - Obtain front loading washers and dryers, which make laundry chores easier from a wheelchair.
  - Place extra cleaning supplies where they are easily accessed.
  - Use light-weight and long-handled tools which can make cleaning easier.

- *Recreation and leisure adaptations:* After completing work and self-care activities, a large amount of time is devoted to leisure and recreation. If you were physically active before your spinal cord injury, many of these activities may be affected. Often people will find themselves spending more of their time on passive pursuits, such as watching TV or listening to the radio. Though how you did things in the past may be different from how you do things after SCI, there are a wide range of adaptations that can help you resume many of the activities you enjoyed before your injury. See *Leisure and Recreation* for more information.

If you enjoyed spending time outdoors, there are wheelchair accessible tents, campgrounds and fishing piers, as well as adapted fishing and hunting equipment. Every year people with SCI catch fish, shoot deer, participate in archery and many other outdoor activities with adaptive equipment.

Hobbies requiring fine motor skills may not be possible without good hand function. However, a skilled recreational or occupational therapist can help you creatively adapt your favorite interests to your functional abilities. Using a deltoid aid and adapted utensils, a person with a tetraplegia may resume painting or ceramics. With a required increase in physical demands, people with SCI can improve their strength, range of motion and endurance over time through adapted recreational and leisure activities.

Find something you enjoy, work with your therapist, work with your caregivers and see how much you can do. While you must always put safety first, you never know what you are capable of accomplishing until you push yourself to your limits.

Keeping in touch with family and friends is important. Talking on a speakerphone or typing on a computer with a typing stick, writing letters or sending cards using a writing aid can help you stay connected to your circle of family and friends. Building social activities into your routine, such as a regularly scheduled card game or attending local school events, can help keep you involved with your community.

Assistive technology
While any device that helps you do something you would otherwise be unable to do is considered assistive technology, many people reserve this term for high-tech devices that typically involve electricity or electronics. Some familiar examples would include voice-activated computers and adapted video games. Many people with paraplegia can use standard, commercially available technology. However, for a person with tetraplegia, standard devices may be unusable. This is where the high-tech types of assistive technology devices and the services of an assistive technology professional are important.

- *Switches and mounts:* With a clear and consistent voice, you may find speech recognition the fastest and most direct method for controlling assistive technology. Sometimes this is not a practical method and then switches need to be used. There are a wide range of simple switches that can be pressed by a finger, elbow, shoulder or head. There are electronic switches that can detect the slightest movement or muscle twitch, like an eye blink. Others are operated by sipping or puffing into a straw. An assistive technology professional can help you find the right switch and mount, in the most effective location for you, to control assistive technology devices.

- *Electronic aids to daily living (EADL):* Essentially any device that uses electricity can be controlled with an EADL. The handicapped door openers at most public buildings are an example of a commercial EADL and are also available in a residential model. It is similar to having a garage door opener for your house.
  — Any gadget that can be turned on or off, such as a fan or light, can be controlled by an X-10 device, which goes between the outlet and the piece of equipment. Pushing a button on a handheld remote, using a switch with a scanning remote or a computer-based program, sends a radio frequency signal to turn the device on/off or dim lights.
  — For devices that use an infrared remote, like a TV or stereo, there are large button, switch or voice-controlled and computer-based remotes that can be matched to just about anyone's ability.
  — Environmental control units (ECUs) are the most sophisticated types of the EADLs. They can control lights, TVs, stereos, hospital beds, a call for help, operation of a phone and a range of other electronic devices. These have a computer or microprocessor that uses a person's voice to control the piece of equipment directly, or a switch that runs through a menu and selects the device and function the person wants to activate.
- *Computer adaptations:* For someone with a high-level spinal cord injury, a computer may be the most powerful device they will be able to use. For many the Accessibility Options, available through the control panel on your operating system, may provide all the modification you need. For example, you can set up the computer for single finger or typing stick use, operate the mouse with the numeric keypad, turn off or slow down the key repeat function.
  — Several types of software programs can help all computer users. For example, computer users of all ability levels with average cognitive skills may find that an abbreviation ex-

pansion program speeds typing of frequently used words and phrases. If you have trouble typing more than 10 to 15 words per minute, you may want to try a word completion or word prediction program. For those with fair voice control and good cognitive skills, speech recognition can increase typing speeds to over 50 words per minute.

— While you can control the mouse cursor with voice control or switches, for those with limited hand function it is much easier with an alternative to a conventional mouse. There are numerous adapted keyboards and key guards that can be used with a finger or typing stick to control the mouse through the numeric keypad. However, most people find trackballs, optical or head pointers are a more effective way to control the cursor. There are also switch interfaces that let you to use any switch to control the mouse buttons. These and a wide range of other hardware adaptations can increase computer productivity for a person with limited hand function and enable him or her to return to school or productive employment.

- *Communication equipment:* While pressing the tiny buttons on a cell phone or handheld phone can be difficult for people with no hand impairment, it can be impossible for someone who has tetraplegia. Fortunately, there are several options available, from large button and scanning phones, to switch and voice operated cell phones. In the hospital people are grateful for having a nurse call switch and a nurse to answer when emergencies arise. At home you can use personal pagers or Lifeline to call for help. For people who must use a ventilator to breathe, there are many alternative and supplemental communication devices that can be operated by keyboard, touch screen, or even eye-gaze, enabling him or her to communicate with others when they are not able to talk using their own voice.

You are not alone in facing the many challenges following a spinal cord injury. There are thousands of health care professionals with specific expertise in spinal cord injury rehabilitation, as well as occupational, recreational, speech and physical therapists with specialized knowledge in assistive technology. There are more than 22,000 assistive devices listed on the Abledata website www.abledata.com, because others before you needed someone to invent something to help them do what they wanted to do.

If there is something you want to do but are unable, then there is probably an assistive technology device that can help you. Talk to your health care provider, therapist or other health care team member and ask them to direct you to an assistive technology professional that can help you find and learn to use the device you need.

THE AMERICANS WITH DISABILITIES ACT OF 1990

The Americans with Disabilities Act (ADA) of 1990 is the most comprehensive legislation ever enacted to protect the rights of people with disabilities. The law references more than 20 other federal laws and regulations, which affect a wide range of activities and services. It also promotes access by eliminating architectural barriers and prohibiting discrimination against qualified persons with disabilities.

The purpose of this material is to inform you about the Americans with Disabilities Act. The ADA has several sections, called "titles."

Employment

Title I prohibits job discrimination against a qualified person with a disability. When the law took effect in July 1992, it applied to most employers with 25 or more employees. In July 1994, coverage was extended to most employers with 15 or more employees.

A "qualified" person with a disability is a person who, with or without reasonable accommodations, can perform the functions needed to do the job that person holds or desires. Under Title I, employers, labor unions and employment agencies may not discriminate against such people in job application procedures, hiring, advancement, discharge, wages and benefits, training, or other terms and conditions of employment.

Reasonable accommodations

Employers are required to make reasonable accommodations for qualified persons with disabilities. The definition of "reasonable accommodations" depends specifically on the person, disability, job and employer.

Such accommodations may include:
- Adapting existing facilities to be readily accessible and usable by persons with disabilities
- Modification of work schedules
- Reassignment to a vacant position

- Acquisition or modification of equipment or devices
- Modification of examinations, training materials, or other programs
- Provision of qualified readers or interpreters

Employers may need to spend money on their buildings or on equipment for these changes. However, the ADA provides that employers need not make changes that will result in "undue hardship" on the operation or employer's business. "Undue hardship" can be defined according to many factors, including the nature and cost of the changes needed, the overall financial resources of the employer, its size, and the number of employees.

Public Services

The requirements of Title II are technical and lengthy. They focus on transportation (buses and rail systems, but not aircraft or public school transportation) accessibility for people with disabilities. Most of the rules are related to wheelchair access.

Public Accommodations

Title III prohibits discrimination against people with disabilities in public accommodation. "Public accommodation" includes a broad list of businesses such as:
- Hotels, motels
- Restaurants, bars
- Theaters, concert halls, stadiums
- Auditoriums, convention centers
- Stores (grocery and department stores, shopping centers, bakeries)
- Service establishments (laundromats, banks, travel agencies, gas stations, hospitals)
- Professional office buildings (doctor's or lawyer's office)
- Museums, libraries, galleries
- Amusement parks, zoos, parks
- Schools, colleges
- Day care centers, senior citizen centers
- Gyms, health spas, bowling alleys

People cannot be discriminated against on the basis of disability. The law indicates that persons with disabilities should have "full and equal enjoyment of the goods, services, facilities, privileges, advantages or accommodations." Public business must make reasonable changes to policies, practices or procedures, or provide auxiliary aids and services as long as these do not cause undue hardship, as previously defined. They must also remove architectural and communication barriers where "readily achievable." If barrier removal is not readily achievable, businesses must provide alternative access.

"Readily achievable" means "easily accomplishable and able to be carried out without much difficulty or expense." The decision depends on the specific circumstances. Certain private clubs and religious organizations are exempt.

Telecommunication

Title IV requires the telecommunications industry to provide Telecommunications Devices of the Deaf (TDD) and other relay services to persons with disabilities. The services are to be available not only to people with hearing or speech disabilities, but also to people with standard telephones who wish to call someone who uses a TDD.

Miscellaneous

Title V contains miscellaneous information. It sets out general regulations for construction, exempts insurance underwriting from the law, prohibits retaliation and coercion, describes rights to attorneys' fees, and outlines other requirements of the law.

The ADA is a complex law that affects many aspects of life for people with disabilities. Talk to a member of your health team for more information regarding the American with Disabilities Act.

Additional Information

Research and Clinical Trials

Following spinal cord injury, many patients and families begin to search for treatments available to repair their own or their loved one's damaged spinal cord. Although no cure is available yet, advances have been made in the science of spinal cord repair and treatments to improve function. As new treatments emerge, it is helpful to understand some basic research concepts before participating in any clinical research trials. Find information from reliable sources and seek the opinion of your primary or SCI-specific health care provider before enrolling in any study.

The purpose of this section is to provide you with some information regarding clinical research trials and unproven clinical treatments, as well as benefits and risks of research studies, and available resources.

Clinical Research Trials versus Unproven Clinical Treatments

The United States Food and Drug Administration (FDA), is committed to protecting persons participating in clinical trials in the United States. They ensure that new drugs and treatments are safe and effective. The FDA requires extensive preclinical testing and reviews proposed research plans before allowing humans to participate in trials. These regulatory requirements are not consistent throughout the world and therefore, unproven treatments may be offered in countries other than the United States.

Clinical research trials in the United States are registered at www.clinicaltrials.gov and have extensive animal investigations that show strong repeatable effects prior to human involvement. The clinical trial design compares a group of patients receiving the experimental treatment to others receiving an alternative treatment.

Clinical trials have four phases that must occur to qualify as a treatment for human patients.

- *Phase 1:* Goal is to find out if the treatment is safe. This phase includes studying a small number of patients who receive the treatment at a low dose to evaluate for side effects.
- *Phase 2:* Goal is to determine positive effects of the treatment by comparing patients receiving the treatment with a control group.
- *Phase 3:* Goal is to demonstrate a useful effect and to monitor side effects. This phase requires a much larger number of patients. Therefore, multiple clinics are involved, comparing patients with experimental treatment to a control group.
- *Phase 4:* Goal is to determine therapeutic safety, drug interactions, contraindications, continued optimization of dose, and additional information on risks, benefits and optimal use. These studies are conducted after the drug or intervention has been approved and marketed to test the drug for new uses.

Unproven clinical treatments are just as the name indicates, unproven. These treatments are often offered without the safety and the efficacy testing that is required in clinical research trials. Although many patients and families are anxiously seeking a cure, participation in unproven treatments may cause harm and generally are not covered by insurance. Unfortunately, it can be difficult to tell when treatments are unproven. Many web sites make claims that their treatments are proven and imply endorsements that are not accurate. Before participating in any "cutting edge treatment" consider obtaining one or two second opinions from people that are independent of the group offering treatment.

Benefits versus Risks of Research Studies

Benefits of participating in well designed SCI research studies include:

- Playing an active role in your health care
- Gaining access to new research treatments before they are widely available
- Helping others by contributing to medical research

Risks of participating in SCI research studies include:

- Adverse health effects
- Participation in other SCI clinical research trials may be limited or disallowed
- Treatment may not be effective
- Time commitment may be significant

Considerations before participating in a research study

The decision to participate in a research study is entirely yours. You can stop your participation at any time. The research health care team or the study sponsor can end your participation at any time if it is in your best interest, if you do not follow the study rules, or the study is stopped.

You should know as much as possible about any study you partici-pate in. In addition, you should feel comfortable asking the health care research team any questions about the study, the care you can expect while participating in the study and the cost involved. Federal rules require that informed consent must be obtained and properly documented before a participant is enrolled in a study. In most cases, the participant must sign and date a detailed informed consent form.

The following questions might be helpful for you to discuss with the research health care team. Some of the answers to these ques-tions may be found in the informed consent document.

- What is the purpose of the study?
- Why do researchers believe the new treatment being tested may be effective? Has it been studied before?
- Who is going to be in the study?
- What kind of tests and treatments are involved?
- Are there treatments other than the experimental one that are currently available for my injury or illness?
- How do the possible risks and benefits in the study compare with my current treatment?
- How long will my participation in the trial last?
- Will hospitalization be required?
- Will results of the study be provided to me?
- Who will pay for the treatment?
- Will I be reimbursed for other expenses?
- What type of long term follow up care is part of the study?
- Who will be in charge of my care?
- How will I know the treatment is working?
- How might this trial affect my daily life?
- Who do I contact with questions?
- Could my condition or my health get worse after this treat-ment?
- What is the maximum level of recovery I might see after this treatment?
- How will potential benefits be measured?

- Is there preclinical evidence that demonstrates the treatment to be beneficial?
- Have the preclinical findings been replicated? If so, is there agreement among researchers that this treatment meets targeted results and will improve my functional outcome?
- Is this study registered as a clinical trial with an appropriate qualified regulatory body?
- Will my participation in this study limit my participation in other spinal cord injury clinical trials?

Available Resources

There are many web sites, articles and news releases that are dedicated to research for SCI. Consult your primary or SCI-specific health care provider when considering enrollment in a clinical research trial or if you have questions regarding such studies.

Many resources listed below can be found on the Internet through your favorite search engine of through the Internet address listed. Except for information and resources supplied by Mayo Clinic, Mayo does not endorse any of the following organizations or resources. This list is not comprehensive.

- National Institute of Neurological Disorders and Stroke: www.ninds.nih.gov/disorders/sci/detail_sci.htm
- Christopher and Dana Reeve Foundation: www.christopher reeve.org
- National Spinal Cord Injury Association: www.spinalcord.org
- Paralyzed Veterans of America (PVA): www.pva.org
- Miami Project to Cure Paralysis: www.themiamiproject.org
- National Institute on Disability and Rehabilitation Research (NIDRR): www.ed.gov/about/offices/list/osers/nidrr
- Morton Cure Paralysis Fund: www.mcpf.org
- The Paralysis Project of America: www.paralysisproject.org
- International Campaign for Cures of Spinal Cord Injury Paralysis: www.icord.org
- Clinical trials: www.clinicaltrials.gov
- Model Spinal Cord Injury System Dissemination Center: www.mscisdisseminationcenter.org
- National Center for the Dissemination of Disability Research: www.ncddr.org

Resources for Those Living with a Disability

This section provides information about resources available to you and how these resources may help you plan for the future. Ask a member of your health care team if you have questions about this information or for additional information and resources.

In addition to the resources listed below, information about living with a disability is available through your local library, bookstores, support groups and the Internet. Except for information and resources supplied by Mayo Clinic, Mayo does not endorse any of the following organizations or resources. This list is not comprehensive.

Many resources listed below can be found on the Internet through your favorite search engine or through the Internet addresses listed. Ask to talk to a medical social worker for more information about how to contact these resources. If other contacts (besides your medical social worker) are available for any of the following resources, it is noted.

Internet resources

www.mayoclinic.org
www.mayoclinic.com
www.healthfinder.gov
www.medlineplus.gov

Americans with Disabilities Act (ADA)

The Americans with Disabilities Act (ADA) protects the rights of people with disabilities and affects a wide range of activities and services.

www.ada.gov

215

Financial resources

Getting your financial affairs in order as soon as possible after an injury or illness is an important part of planning for your future. During your rehabilitation, ask to meet with a medical social worker specializing in rehabilitation. This social worker may help you and your family in many areas of adjustment, including financial planning. The following financial resources may be available to you.

Social Security Disability Insurance (SSDI)

If you have worked and paid into Social Security, you and your dependents may be eligible for cash benefits. To qualify, you have to have paid enough into the Social Security system and you have to be considered legally disabled by the Social Security Administration. Ask your Social Security Administration office for more information at www.ssa.gov/disability.

Supplemental Security Income (SSI)

Supplemental Security Income assures a minimum monthly income to people who are considered to be legally disabled, elderly or blind. To qualify, you must meet financial eligibility requirements since this is a need-based program. Some people are eligible for both SSDI and SSI. Check with the Social Security Administration office for more information at www.ssa.gov/disability.

Medicare

Medicare is a federal health insurance program for people 65 or older who are receiving Social Security retirement benefits. People younger than 65 who receive Social Security disability benefits also may be eligible. Individuals, who are deemed to be disabled under Social Security Disability for more than two consecutive years, are automatically enrolled in Medicare. This federally funded insurance program covers a wide range of medical needs, including hospital stays and medical care. For more information: www.medicare.gov.

Under some circumstances home health care, equipment, ambulance transportation and other benefits are covered. Ask your Social Security Administration office for more information on this program.

State welfare programs

Your local county Department of Social Services may be a resource for several federal and state funded programs. Services may include:
- Medicaid (Medical Assistance)
- Food stamps
- General assistance

To find out if you are eligible for these services and programs and to apply, you or a family member will need to complete an application in the county where you live.

Veterans Administration (VA) and Veterans Services (VS)

Disabled veterans may be eligible for benefits including hospital stays, medical treatment, medications, educational programs, pensions and other federal programs. A Veterans Service office is located in each county. Call your local Veterans Service representative for information and assistance with applying or you may find information at www.va.gov

Workers' compensation

If you have been injured on the job, you may be eligible for workers' compensation. This state-regulated program pays medical costs and other benefits to workers who have been injured on the job. To be eligible, you must have been employed by an organization that is covered by workers' compensation. Check with your employer or the personnel office of your place of employment for more information.

Vocational Rehabilitation Services

You may be eligible for aid through Vocational Rehabilitation Services (VRS), a federal and state funded agency, which typically has many offices throughout most states. This agency helps people who have disabilities with medical and rehabilitation evaluation and re-training, which assists in a return to suitable employment. Some states have funds available through this agency for attendant care, changes in your home and other services. Ask your local VRS office for additional information. More information can be found at:
- Office of Disability: www.ed.gov/about/offices/list/osers/rsa/new.html
- Office of Disability Employment Policy (ODEP): www.dol.gov/odep
- Job Accommodation Network (JAN): www.jan.wvu.edu

Services for the Blind and Visually Handicapped

For people who have a significant visual loss, the Services for the Blind and Visually Handicapped provides services similar to those of the Vocational Rehabilitation Services. It is funded by state and federal funds.

Personal health insurance

Insurance coverage varies greatly among different insurance policies, depending on the contract of the individual policy. To confirm your benefits, call your hospital account representative or insurance representative. Discuss insurance concerns with your medical social worker.

Accessibility resources

Changes in housing, accessibility, and assistive technology

Members of the rehabilitation team, especially the occupational and physical therapists, may be available to assess your living arrangements and check needed housing adaptations. This evaluation may include a visit to your home. Other people with physical disabilities who have been through the experience of making changes in their homes can also provide valuable information about the process, as well as show the results of these changes.

To finance these changes, consider such resources as workers' compensation benefits. If you were injured in an automobile accident, check your automobile insurance coverage. Also, Vocational Rehabilitation Services may be a possible resource for limited changes, depending on the agency's resources. Grants or loans for changes may also be available in your area. To receive financial help through any outside agency, approval for changes must be obtained from the funding agency before beginning any changes. Contact the specific agency for additional information.

Information regarding assistive technology can be found at:
- Spinal Peer Information Library on Technology: www.scipilot.com
- Center for Assistive Technology and Environmental Access: www.assistivetech.net

Education resources

Hospital-bound and home-bound tutoring

Hospital-bound tutoring is available for people under 21 who have not graduated from high school. After leaving the hospital, students

who cannot return to the classroom or their parents should call the local school principal or superintendent of schools to request more educational services. Another educational resource
for parents is the Parent Advocacy Coalition for Educational Rights (PACER): www.pacer.org.

General Education Development (GED)

People who have not earned a high school diploma may do so by successfully completing the General Education Development (GED) examination. Most colleges, universities and employers recognize this diploma. You can get information on GED testing from your State Department of Education. You may need tutoring before a GED examination. Under some circumstances, the tutoring may be arranged during your hospital stay. After leaving the hospital, you can find more information on this program through the guidance department of your local high school, local adult education centers, a local community or junior college, or Vocational Rehabilitation Services.

College education

According to law, colleges must make reasonable accommodations for all students, disabled or able-bodied. This includes accessibility, parking and other special services. Many colleges have special programs to help people with disabilities complete a college education. Talk to your college of interest for additional information.

Driver training

Many people with a disability may be eager to return to an active life in their communities by returning to driving. Some people with a disability, such as a spinal cord injury, cannot drive as before. He or she must learn to rely on hand controls when driving. Driver training with hand controls for people with disabilities may be available during your rehabilitation. Contact driver education schools regarding hand control training.

Advocacy resources

SSI Disability Advocacy

Outreach services employs trained advocates and experienced disability attorneys to facilitate application for Social Security Disability enrollment. This program is for residents of MN only.

Consumer education resources

Additional consumer educational resources for persons with spinal cord injury, including information on autonomic hyperreflexia, bowel management and depression, are available from Paralyzed

Veterans of America at www.pva.org. Or, you can search "consortium for spinal cord medicine" in your web browser to find a variety of printable and downloadable guides. Other educational resources include:

- American Paraplegia Society: www.apssci.org
- American Spinal Injury Association: www.asia-spinalinjury.org
- Internatinal Spinal Cord Society: www.iscos.org.uk
- National Institute on Disability and Rehabilitation: www.ed.gov/about/offices/list/osers/nidrr
- National Rehabilitation Center: www.naric.com
- National Spinal Cord Injury Association: www.spinalcord.org
- Spinal Cord Injury Information Network: www.spinalcord.uab. edu
- Spinal Cord Injury Resource Center: www.spinalinjury.net
- United Spinal Assocation: www.unitedspinal.org

Personal resources

Psychological support

A disability or injury can challenge a person's ability to cope with his or her emotions. Depression, anger, confusion, self-doubt, anxiety and many other emotions may surface while learning to adjust to a new disability. These feelings are normal reactions to major losses and to stress. Over time and with support, you can work through these feelings. Counseling provides a supportive, safe environment in which to explore your feelings, take risks and consider alternatives.

Psychological support is available to you through psychiatrists, psychologists, clinical social workers, rehabilitation counselors, clergy and mental health clinics, as well as other members of the rehabilitation team. The support of your family is perhaps the most important part of your adjustment. In addition, peer visitors who have learned to live with disabilities, are also available to you to share their experiences and practical information with you.

Psychologists who are specifically trained to work with persons with disabilities are called rehabilitation psychologists. They can be located at the American Board of Rehabilitation Psychology at: www.abrp.org.

Centers for Independent Living

Some states have set up Centers for Independent Living. These are consumer-oriented agencies serving people who have a variety of disabilities. The following services may be available:

- Referral to community resources
- Financial information and counseling
- Information about accessible and affordable housing
- Information on personal care assistants as well as management training, which may assist with becoming a successful employer of a personal care assistant
- Information on peer visitors; people who have learned to live successfully with a disability and can share experiences with people who have similar disabilities
- Support for people who are having trouble meeting their needs in their community

For information about the National Council for Independent Living, go to: www.ncil.org or Independent Living USA, at: www.ilusa.com.

Personal care assistant

Some people with a new injury or illness need a personal care assistant after leaving the rehabilitation unit. A personal care assistant is a person who helps you to do things that you cannot physically do yourself. Some personal care assistants can be obtained with the help of Centers for Independent Living. When such centers are not available, other sources may be used, which may include:
- College bulletin boards and placement offices
- Friends who have attendants
- Local newspapers including college papers
- Employment offices
- Public Health Department
- Leads from friends

During your rehabilitation, you may learn techniques for hiring, training and contracting a personal care assistant.

Home health care

After leaving the hospital, some people may need someone from a home health agency to come into their home to provide limited nursing care. Most communities have at least one home health agency that can provide intermittent care at home, either on a short-term or a long-term basis.

Travel and Recreation

Travel and recreational resources are available at:
- Access-Able Travel Source: www.access-able.com
- Disabled Sports USA: www.dsusa.org

Legal representation

People who have had a disability from an accident may wish to call an attorney of their choice, to become informed of their rights and to pursue compensation. If you need legal advice or help in choosing a private attorney, call your local county bar association.

Tax information

By claiming certain exclusions and deductions provided by law, people with a disability may save money on federal income tax. Many things that help a person with a disability to function better, may qualify as a medical deduction. In most cases, attendant care services are tax deductible. For more information and help with your income tax, call a certified public accountant.

Addresses and telephone numbers
_____

_____

_____

Your local Social Security office
_____

_____

_____

Medical social worker
_____

_____

_____

Other
_____

_____

_____

Glossary

This word list defines some terms that you may not know which were used in this book.

Autonomic hyperreflexia (dysreflexia): A potentially life-threatening rise in blood pressure which occurs in people with spinal cord injuries above T6. The cause is painful stimuli below the level of injury.

Constipation: Infrequent or difficult passage of hard stool.

Cystitis: Inflammation or infection of the urinary bladder.

Cystoscopy: A procedure done with a small instrument (cystoscope) which has a light on the end. The cystoscope is passed through the urethra into the bladder. The bladder wall can be viewed and procedures can be done using this instrument.

Decubitus ulcer: See pressure ulcer.

Detrusor muscles: Muscles that form the wall of the bladder.

Diaphragm: Dome-shaped muscle separating the chest from the abdomen. It is a major muscle involved in breathing.

Diarrhea: Passing of more than three loose, watery stools a day.

Digital stimulation: Gently moving a well-lubricated, gloved finger in the rectum to cause a bowel movement by reflex.

Dysfunction: Not functioning normally.

Dysreflexia: See autonomic hyperreflexia.

Dyssynergia: Uncoordinated contraction of the bladder muscle and sphincter.

Ejaculation: Expulsion of semen from the penis as a result of stimulation.

Electroejaculation: Electrical stimulation applied by a probe inserted into the rectum to cause an ejaculation.

Embolus: A blood clot or foreign body within a blood vessel that travels in the bloodstream until it becomes lodged in a smaller vessel.

External "condom catheter": Urinary collection device for men, in which a condom is connected to a bag by tubing.

Flaccid: Soft, limp, without muscle tone.

Heterotopic ossification: Bone formation in soft tissue, usually near the joints.

Incontinence: Unexpected and/or uncontrolled passage of urine and/or stool.

Neurogenic bladder: Loss of normal control of bladder function due to spinal cord, peripheral nerve or brain damage.

Neurogenic bowel: Loss of normal control of bowel function due to spinal cord, peripheral nerve or brain damage.

Paralysis: A condition in which a person is unable to move his or her muscles when attempting to do so.

Paraparesis: Incomplete paralysis which may involve the trunk, legs and pelvic organs.

Paraplegia: Complete paralysis of the legs, parts of the trunk and pelvic organs.

Pelvic floor muscles: A group of muscles at the base of the pelvis, which help support the bladder, urethra, rectum and (in women) vagina and uterus.

Peristalsis: Automatic wavelike movement of the intestine.

Pressure ulcer: An open sore that forms on the skin due to prolonged pressure.

Quadriparesis/tetraparesis: Incomplete paralysis of all four limbs and the trunk.

Quadriplegia/tetraplegia: Paralysis involving all or part of the arms, trunk, legs and pelvic organs.

Reflux: Backward movement of body fluids, such as urine returning from the bladder into the ureters and kidneys.

Spastic: Involuntary tightening or movement of muscles.

Sphincter: Circular muscles at an orifice that upon contraction, close the opening. The body has several sphincter muscles, including those at the anus, bladder and opening to the stomach from the esophagus.

Spinal canal: The canal through the vertebrae where the spinal cord is located.

Spinal cord: The part of the central nervous system that connects the brain with the peripheral nerves. It extends from the base of the brain to the small of the back inside the spinal canal.

Tetraplegia: See quadriplegia.

Thrombosis: Development of a blood clot attached to the inside of a blood vessel.

Trachea: Tubelike structure that connects the mouth and lungs; also known as the windpipe.

Index

Note: page numbers followed by *f* or *t* indicate that the citation may be found in a figure or table.